Dr. John R. Christopher

Herbal Home Health Care

Printing Errors

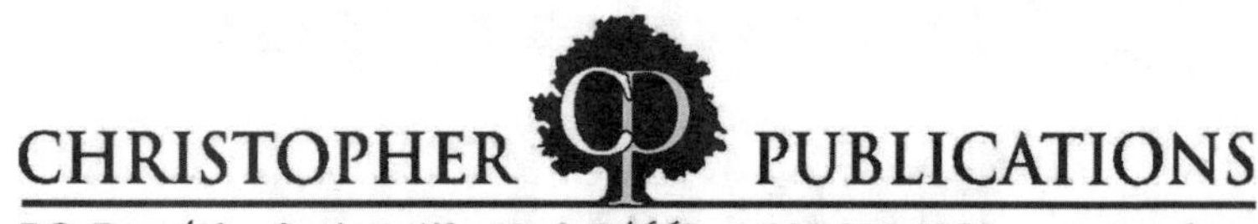

P.O. Box 412 • Springville, Utah 84663 1-800-372-8255 • www.snh.cc

ISBN #1-879436-03-5

Reprinted 1998, Updated and Reprinted 2004
Cover design by Nathan Jaynes

Printed in the United States of America
by Christopher Publications.

The information contained in this book is not intended to be used to diagnose or prescribe in any way. This book is not meant to take the place of advice from a qualified health care practitioner.

FOREWORD

My life style, as I went through childhood, may have been the main reason I have written this book on childhood diseases. My lot in life was to have been born sickly, and so I had the misfortune to have contracted nearly all childhood diseases.

This sickly childhood of mine gave me a desire to see better health in children, our own and others. I didn t actually know a good healthy day throughout my childhood and, for that matter, until I was past thirty-five years old. Over the years much trial and error was used to keep me alive and in motion.

As the years continued on, the desire to help myself and others grew strong within me. In my twenties I began to experiment with diet and in building up my body, and wrote a little book entitled *Just What Is the Word of Wisdom?* I then studied at schools where I learned about herbs and diet. The first of these schools was the Dominion Herbal College in Vancouver, B.C. Here I received my Master Herbalist (M.H.) degree as an herbal doctor. The next step was getting my degree as a naturopathic physician from the School of Drugless Therapy in Iowa. I next studied under Dr. Edward Shook at the Los Angeles Herbal Institute to receive my herbal pharmacist degree.

After starting to assist people, young and old, to regain their health I began to realize how much sickness was present. For over thirty-six years now, it has been my pleasure to see thousands of people healed by the simple procedures of the natural routine.

In this book it is our desire to pass on many of the aids we have used over the years and to tell it in a simple form so the layman may glean value from this work.

In appreciation I would like to mention a few of the fine folks that have given me help to write this and other books and articles.

As is commonly known, an author who is active and busy does not always have time, or sometimes the knack, for using good grammar alone. Many authors have ghost writers and pay editing and research, as they (busy doctors, church leaders, political heads, etc.) cannot take time for close detail work and keep up the demands placed upon them in other activities.

I travel and lecture to well over a hundred major cities each year. If my many hours of lecturing could be put into books, it would take an entire staff of assistants to correct my English, sentence structure, etc. With the books I have written, magazine articles, newsletters, interviews, etc., all my writing has to be reviewed for error. It seems I have the ability to speak and lecture (or the gift of gab), but when I take a pen into my hand I write poor grammar. It must be my pen!

The first person I turn my work over to is my dear wife, Della. She has been a great blessing to me, because she sees my glaring mistakes. She gives me wonderful suggestions to aid in my writings and I must say I would be lost without her. (One of her first suggestions: Don t start every sentence with a preposition!) (Bet you guessed it, I am a very lucky man.)

At times a lot of manuscripts are are being worked on at the same time and we need some extra help. Over the years we have had excellent assistance from some well qualified people. One person I d like to mention is Cathy Gileadi. She has spent a lot of time in doing research for my books and articles and has performed other much needed tasks. As a good example, I will give her a number of rare old books from my library and ask her to add any new material on a certain herb or subject that I have not used before. Sometimes she will do an index or correct my (at times) unsavory sentence structure.

These folks helping me now in our writings are quite different from one experience I had a number of years ago. I had been in my present occupation for approximately 30 years when I allowed a college student who could not afford my lectures to assist me in transcribing my taped lectures and also researching new material. In return, the student attended my classes free of charge and obtained other knowledge on herbs. The student was later paid a wage for his work. Unfortunately, later on, this student claimed authorship to those lectures.

We must have the bitter to appreciate the sweet, and that is why I am so happy with the people who are helping me at this time.

Our typist, Sharon Ann Bird, is a jewel who works overtime to rush through articles that are on quick call and deadline materials for the publishers. Always she is there smiling and ready to go to work.

I am very grateful to all of those who have helped me in my writings, named or unnamed. I am especially grateful to our five children John, Ruth, David, Janet, and Steve who have been so much help, and who have stuck with their father through thick and thin (persecutions, ups and downs, etc.) these many years. Our son David, who travels a lot with me, and his wife Fawn, who does my correspondence, have been especially helpful.

Even though at times the world reviles, my family and friends make me a blessed man indeed, and I am deeply grateful for such blessings.

Dr. John Raymond Christopher

This book is dedicated to Dr. Christopher s twenty-four grandchildren and twenty-six great grandchildren.

Table of Contents

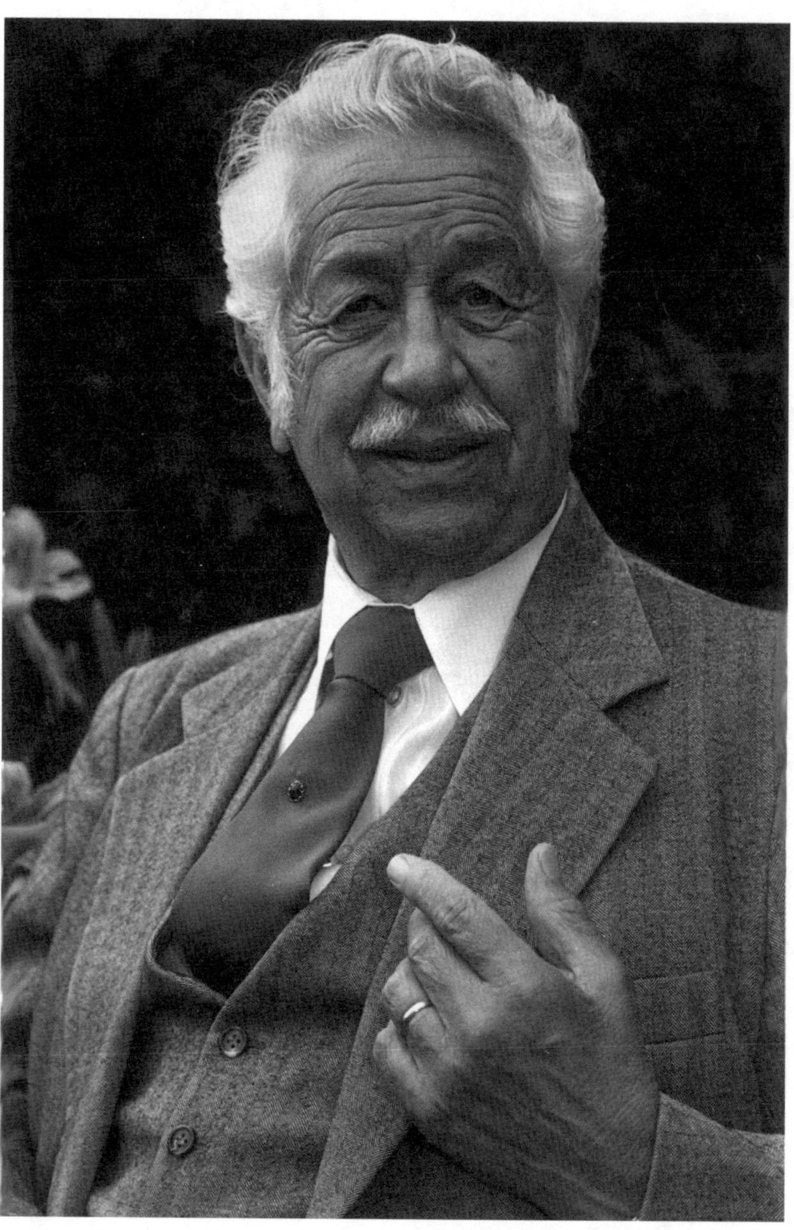

INTRODUCTION

We are going to talk about the subject of childhood diseases. Just when should we be concerned about weaknesses in the child s body, which make it susceptible to disease? The time we start preparing to build a strong immune system in the child is many months before conception. If, however, that is too late and the child is here and sick at this time, we have to work on the present cause; but this effort could have been avoided had we started a few generations back. We are told that the sins of the parents will be passed on to the children up to the third and fourth generations. These are sins of commission or omission. In most cases, thank goodness, it is the sin of omission because we did not know better.

Over the past several generations, catering to our taste buds has pulled us away from eating wholesome foods. We have now switched over to the processed merchandise (I hate to call it food); to not only pamper the taste bud, but eliminate a lot of time in food preparation.

Through processing our food we have depleated it of many minerals, vitamins, natural fiber, etc., and have wound up with junk materials that are not fit for man or beast. With each generation that pulls away from God-given wholesome food, we add insult to injury by weakening our children, who pass the same weakenesses on to their children. As our society becomes more modern the problem gets even worse as more inorganic additives (and in many instances cancer causing preservatives) are being used. It is almost like a new challenge. Let s preserve the food stuffs, not the people!

A child could live without the fear of sickness of crippling disease if he had, in the beginning, a good strong body. Disease germs are scavengers and can live only on weak wasting-away cells, excess mucus, and toxic conditions. Never can germs thrive in a healthy and clean cell structure.

Prior to marriage is the time to set the stage for the healthy offsprings to follow. Prepare the parent-to-be to live for abundant health so the will be able to have healthy children.

If all parents-to-be would follow the mucusless diet, then the start for a healthy new generation would appear on the horizon and the thousand years of millennial peace would dawn onto a new race of healthy disease-free people.

CHAPTER ONE

Health for Prospective Parents

If one has been living on the mucusless diet and is now expecting a new healthy child, remember, faith without works is not the proper way to go. To carry on the good works of proper diet and preparation for the new mother-to-be, one should include additional aids to purify her body, in order to pass on good health to the expected child.

Besides keeping away from mucus-forming and toxic food stuffs, she should also be using special foods and wholistic procedures to assist the new one coming, and to give her an easier time during pregnancy and delivery.

THE MOTHER-TO-BE

One of the best herbal foods is red raspberry leaf tea. This is made by using a heaping teaspoon of red raspberry leaves to each cup of hot steam-distilled water, or one ounce of the herbs (two heaping tablespoons, approximately) to each pint of distilled water. Never let the tea boil, but pour the boiling water over the herbs and then steep fifteen or twenty minutes in a warm place, strain and drink. It is best to drink three or more cups a day of this tea during the entire pregnancy. It is a pleasant-tasting tea and is also an anti-nausea remedy.

To learn a little more about red raspberry leaf tea, let s go to a good source to see what values it carries. We quote from Agricultural Research Services: Phytochemical & Ethnobotanical Databases (www.ars-grin.gov/duke/). All nutrients listed are found in the leaf itself.

Alpha-Carotene	Manganese
Alpha-Tocopherol	Niacin
Ascorbic Acid	Pectin
Boron	Phosphorus
Calcium	Potassium
Chromium	Riboflavin

Fiber	Selenium
Iron	Silica
Magnesium	Thiamin
Malic Acid	Zinc

The following description of red raspberry comes from the *School of Natural Healing* (by Dr. John R. Christopher, Christopher Publications):

Identifying Characteristics:
Erect and freely branched, 3-6 feet high, glaucous, spiny (covered with small, straight and slender prickles).

Leaves:
Pinnate, stalked, 2 pairs of ovate leaflets and a larger terminal leaflet, rounded base, double serrate margins, abruptly pointed at apex, pale green above, grayish white beneath with ap pressed felted hairs, 2 1/2 - 3 1/2 inches long, 2 - 3 inches broad.

Flowers:
Small, white pendulous (hanging), clusters of five, cup-shaped corolla.

Fruit:
Red berry, globular cluster of 20-30 small, rounded and succu lent drupelets, numerous hairs, fleshly, red juice (sweet, pleas ant, acidulous), small stony endocarps (pits).

Taste: Astringent.

Parts used: Leaves, also root, bark, fruit.

Therapeutic action:
Astringent, tonic, stimulant, alterative, stomachic, anti-emetic,

parturient, hemostatic, cathartic, antiseptic, anti-abortive, anti-gonorrheal, anti-leucorrheal, antimalarial. Fruit: Mildly laxative, esculent, antacid, parturient, refrigerant.

Red raspberry is a great agent for cleansing a canker condition of the mucous membranes in the alimentary tract, leaving the tissue toned. In pregnancy the infusion, when taken regularly, will quiet premature pains and will produce a safe, speedy and easy delivery. Raspberry leaves stimulate, tone and regulate (both the leaves and fruit are high in citrate of iron which is the active alterative, blood-making, astringent and contractive agent for the reproductive area) before and during childbearing, assisting contractions and checking hemorrhage during labor, relieving after-pains, then strengthening, cleansing and enriching the milk of the mother in the post-delivery period. The tea is a valuable and effective agent for female menstrual problems, decreasing the menstrual flow without stopping it abruptly. Raspberry leaves are soothing and toning to the stomach and bowels, with healing action to sore mouths, sore throats, nausea, aphtha, stomatitis, diabetes, diarrhea and dysentery. They are especially valuable in stomach and bowel complaints of children.

Medicinal uses:
Constipation, nausea, diarrhea, dysentery, diabetes, pregnancy, uterine hemorrhage, parturition, uterine cramps, labor pains, cholera infantum, leucorrhea, prolapsus uteri, prolapsus ani, hemorrhoids, dyspepsia, vomiting, colds, fevers, intestinal flu, bowel complaint, thrush, relaxed sore throat, ophthalmia, sore mouth, sore throat, spongy gums, ulcers, wounds, gonorrhea.

Preparation:
Decoction, fluid extract, infusion, powder, tincture.

There are many more pages in this volume on formulas and many other data, but what we have shown here is enough to demonstrate to you a great pre-remedy as well as a body builder for the baby to be. Other herbal books such as Kloss *Back to Eden* and Meyer s *The Herbalist* also sing praises to red raspberry leaf tea.

Before and during the pregnancy it is always extremely important to see that the reproductive organs are functioning properly, and producing the correct amounts of hormones and estrogens.

If the female organs are in a questionable condition, before and during pregnancy, and also in the post-delivery period, it is helpful to use our Female Reproductive Formula (Nu-Fem) an herbal food to strengthen and rebuild the entire reproductive area. The Hormonal Changease Formula can also be used to assist in supplying needed hormones and estrogens in the correct amount. The human body is computerized to a point that it will take the different types of estrogens and hormones it needs from any food and easily discard the ones not used. These herbs can not only be accepted into the body, but assimilated when needed and eliminated when not required. Many inorganic drugs can be accepted into the body but assimilated only in small amounts. The rest of the prescription, being inorganic and of a low vibration, cannot be eliminated with ease and lies in weakened areas, accumulating to cause side-effects and after-effects as time progresses.

The Female Reproductive Formula (Nu-Fem). This is an amazing combination of herbs to aid in rebuilding a malfunctioning reproductive system (uterus, ovaries, fallopian tubes, etc.). Over the years herbalists and patients have seen painful menstruations, heavy flowing, cramps, irregularity, etc., that have been relieved by using this aid to readjust the malfunctioning areas, resulting in a painless menstrual period, good menstrual timing, and a new outlook on life. The Female Reproductive Formula consists of three parts of goldenseal root and one part of each of the following: blessed thistle, cayenne, cramp bark, false unicorn root, ginger, red raspberry leaves, squaw vine, and uva ursi.

Recommended dosage is one cup of tea or two capsules or tablets morning and evening or three times a day if desired. Take this amount for six days a week as long as required to get desired results. We have seen many severe cases clear up in ninety to one hundred and twenty days after many years of suffering. Some get relief sooner, some take longer, no two cases are alike. This is a food to rebuild malfunctioning female reproductive organs.

The Hormonal Changease Formula (Changease). Here are herbs that aid in developing the hormone and estrogen balance in both female and male. This formula consists of the following herbs: black cohosh, sarsaparilla, ginseng, blessed thistle, licorice root, false unicorn root and squaw vine. Adult suggested amount is one to three number 0 capsules morning and evening, as desired. It is an aid to youth going into puberty, for expecting mothers, postpartum (especially for postpartum depression), as well as for women at the time of menopause.

These two formulas, the Female Reproductive and The Hormonal Changease can be used during the entire time of pregnancy (and also before and following), they are an herbal food like any other food. They are there to be used, if needed, and can do no harm in any way.

If there is yeast infection and or herpes simplex before or during pregnancy, add also the vaginal-rectal bolus (VB) formula and the slant board routine. These are very beneficial and yet are harmless to the mother and child-to-be.

The Slant Board Routine and Yellow Dock Combination. As an aid in prolapsed uterus, bowel, or other organs, to assist in giving relief, make a concentrated tea (simmer down to half its amount) of six parts oak bark, three parts mullein, four parts yellow dock root, three parts walnut bark or leaves, six parts comfrey root, one part lobelia, and three parts marshmallow root. Inject with a syringe (while head down on slant board) 1/4 to 1/2 cup or more into the vagina; or one cup or more into the rectum for prolapsus or hemorrhoid problems and leave in as long as is possible before voiding. Dose suggested is one-fourth to one cup, one or more times in a day. When the tea is injected into the abdominal area, and while on the slant board, knead and massage the pelvic and abdominal area to exercise the muscles, so the herbal tea (food) will be assimilated into the organs.

THE FATHER-TO-BE

We are also giving here an herbal formula for the father-to-be. If his reproductive organs are in a good clean healthy condition, the seed for conception will be an improvement over seed of questionable quality. The slant board routine following the rectal bolus at night, along with the Male Urinary Tract Formula (Prospalate), proper mucusless diet and reproductive organ rebuilding will also be an asset to the future family and another aid in preventing childhood diseases.

Male Urinary Tract Formula: In case of malfunction we suggest this combination to assist the male: one part each of cayenne, ginger, goldenseal root, gravel root or queen of the meadow root, juniper berries, marshmallow root, parsley root or herb, uva ursi leaves, and ginseng. This will dissolve the stones that are in the kidneys, as well as clean out other sedimentation and infection in the prostate. Mix the powders and place in No. 0 capsules and take two or more morning and night, with parsley tea when possible. The Prostate Plus Formula (Prospalmetto) is also a specific formula for prostate health.

MISCARRIAGE

The Anti-Miscarriage Formula: A mother-to-be looks forward to the arrival of the new little one, then one day she panics at the discovery of early spotting and then hemorrhaging. This generally is indicative of miscarriage aborting due to the weakened conditions of the reproductive organs.

Over the years we have seen many of these cases, because parents-to-be have turned away from good nutrition and healthy living practices. So the over-all picture of the human culture is a sad one with more and more heartaches from miscarriage.

We offer you a formula here for those who have indication of aborting. This combination should always be on hand because this emergency can appear so quickly that it is shocking and frightening.

The Anti-Miscarriage Formula: The anti-miscarriage formula consists of these two herbs: false unicorn and lobelia. Unless otherwise specified, teas are always made with one teaspoon of herbs to a cup of distilled water if obtainable. If hemorrhaging starts during pregnancy, stay in bed, use a bed pan when needed, and use 1/2 cup of this tea each 1/2 hour until bleeding stops, then each waking hour for one day, remaining in bed as much as possible, and then three times in a day for three weeks. If bleeding continues instead of decreasing, see a qualified midwife or other health care provider.

This combination of one part false unicorn and one part lobelia, used as explained above, will stop the bleeding if the fetus is in a good healthy condition. If the fetus is dead, in many cases the dead fetus is aborted with ease. Without this help, the fetus, when dead, will rarely abort, lying in the womb and causing infection.

PRENATAL

The **Pre-Natal Formula:** We wish to give you another wonderful formula that is used five or six weeks before delivery time. This formula has both black cohosh and pennyroyal herbs in it, which, according to many, are not to be used during times of pregnancy because they could, it is said, cause miscarriage.

This is not so at this late stage (five or six weeks before delivery). If it were so, how could thousands have used this formula so successfully for many years? No, you need have no fear because of false reports that someone had used pennyroyal or black cohosh alone and miscarriage had occurred. We have never had one case of this verified to us. On the other hand we have received angry calls from promiscuous young people who, after reading that people have said these herbs could cause abortion, had used them for this purpose. These young men had given their unmarried pregnant girlfriends quantities of these herbs but no abortion occurred, so they and the girls were angry because of the supposed failure of the herbs.

We have had a report come to us about a young mother-to-be

for the second time who had never heard of the pre-natal combination. Her previous labor was very severe, lasting around thirty hours. After she became pregnant the second time she heard about this pre-natal combination, she got some, used it the last week before delivery, and cut the labor time down to about four hours. She just recently had her third baby with a very short labor and more ease than she had dreamed possible, after using the pre-natal formula for the last six weeks. Many people believe the change from difficult to easy delivery results from using red raspberry leaf tea (and squaw vine tea) throughout the nine months of pregnancy and using the pre-natal combination during the last six weeks. Of course, one of the most important ways a mother can create a healthy baby is by following the mucusless diet faithfully and then doing periodic three-day cleanses. The Three Day Cleanse should be used at least once each month during pregnancy as well as later, during the time of lactation.

Pre-Natal Formula: Using this tea (or two or three capsules or tablets) morning and evening is an aid in giving elasticity to the pelvic and vaginal area and strengthening the reproductive organs for easier delivery. It should be used only in the last six weeks before time of birth. The herbs used in our pre-natal combination are: squaw vine, holy thistle, black cohosh, pennyroyal, false unicorn, raspberry leaves, and lobelia.

The Herbal Calcium Formula: Another way the mother-to-be can ensure having a healthy child (one that is not a worry because of repeated sicknesses), is to use a good calcium formula during the entire pregnancy and also during the lactation period. There is a good herbal formula that we use which is strictly an assimilable, vegetable (herbal) type combination. It consists of six parts horsetail grass, four parts comfrey root, three parts oat straw and one part lobelia. The horsetail grass is almost pure silica but by biological transmutation, so says renowned scientist Professor Louis C. Kervran, the human body is able to transform the silica molecule into assimilable calcium. To aid this we have a number of trace minerals in the comfrey that speeds up the transformation.

It is a known fact that there is a lack of adequate calcium in the diet of the average adult today. One reason, of course, is the use of processed foods which have been robbed of much of the calcium they originally had. The next cause of calcium deficiency is the use of so much inorganic sugars and starches (the starches turn to sugars). This sugar leaches out calcium from the body of the mother. The fetus is also drawing on the mother s calcium for self preservation. The young mother-to-be then wonders why she has varicose veins (breaking and darkening of veins), loss of teeth, and charlie horses (cramps) and muscle weakness, etc.

This all happens because of a lack of adequate calcium to take care of both the mother-to-be and the forthcoming child. Mother Nature is more concerned with the reproduction than with the one doing the producing. This is the reason the baby will draw from the mother as much calcium and nourishment as it can get, and unless she is following a good diet, both will suffer. When there is plenty of calcium (such as is recommended in the formula) being taken by the mother, the fetus will have an ample supply for good development without robbing the mother s veins, teeth, bone and muscles. When this proper program is followed, the fetus will develop as Mother Nature intended and have a strong, perfect body. The umbilical cord is giving the precious little one just as good a blood transfusion as the mother can supply daily by her nutritional intake (good or poor).

Of course, a proper diet does not include items such as cigarettes, pastries, soft drinks, liquor, or coffee. The process of nutrition continues on after the birth of the baby and the umbilical cord is cut. The blood flow carrying this perfect nutrition changes somewhat, as it is now handled by the mammary glands.

The love felt by a baby nursing at its mother s breast is the love that can change the world. During my years as a doctor, many were the times I have said, This child has been bottle fed, or This child has been nursed at the breast. The difference in the emotional characteristics is easily recognized in the child. Articles in national publication are continually citing the fact that many teenage problems come from bottle-feeding.

As a mother nurses her baby, it is suggested by some authorities that she should sing to it or read to it (good poetry and stories). The little one will absorb this therapeutic assistance, and it will pay off later.

Mother dear, you have carried the baby within you in full security and safety for nine months. When it is born, don t cast it off into a bottle world. Take twice the time (approximately eighteen months), hold it close to you, and during the precious nursing times, both of you rest and love each other. This will help make for a happy, loving, secure child.

NURSING

The baby, as it nurses, is still receiving its daily blood transfusion, because the milk is pure blood with only the red corpuscles eliminated. Each mammal has the ability at birth to make its own red corpuscles. Each mammal has marrow in its bones and additional organs to assist in this procedure. Therefore the mother retains and recycles her red corpuscles within herself, and the baby makes its own red corpuscles, but it needs the food carried by the mother s blood (now milk) to continue its growth. The mother s milk and her blood stream are as good as her diet intake, and this is why she should eat properly in order to feed her precious new baby. The following is a comparison between mother s milk and cow s milk by Gladys B. Caster, M.S.

	Breast Milk	**Cow s Milk**
Water	88.3%	87.3%
Mineral salts	0.2%	0.7%
Protein	1.5%	3.5%
Fat	4.0%	4.0%
Sugar	6.0%	4.5%
Reaction	Alkaline	Acid

This is a comparison between nursing and bottle feeding taken from National Resource Defense Council.

Nursing	Formula (Bottle Feeding)
Milk is clean and practically free from bacteria. It is dispensed at the correct temperature and is inexpensive.	Formula may harbor harmful organisms, must be heated and costs hundreds of dollars each year.
Breast milk provides the baby with immune cells from the mother that coincide with the baby s environment.	Immune cells are not provided in formula. Bottle fed babies are more likely to contract some diseases
The proteins in mother s milk are easy for the baby to digest.	The proteins used in formulas is difficult to digest.
Breast fed babies are less likely to develop ear infections and respiratory problems.	Formula fed babies succumb to ear and respiratory infections more often
Breast feeding helps the mother lose weight and helps return the mother s uterus to its normal shape more quickly. Nursing is also a natural contraceptive.	Formula feeding does none of these things.
Mothers who breast feed are less likely to develop osteoporosis, as well as breast cancer later in life.	Formula feeding offers no health benefits to the mother.
Nursing imparts a greater sense of caring, security, and trust in the child.	Less bonding between mother and child occurs.

The mother s body is so perfectly computerized that her milk changes with the need of the baby. As an example, the first clear liquid coming from the breast the first day or so is considered worthless water by some doctors, and the baby is put onto a formula so it will not starve. This very wonderful clear liquid (called colostrum) is not only the most perfect first food for the new infant, but is also such a great laxative, the powers of which man has never been able to duplicate. With this clear worthless liquid much toxic poison provided by some drug and tobacco using mothers is removed from the baby, to make life easier as it develops into childhood.

The lactation process is a miracle within itself. The new born infant has no gastric juices flowing until it cuts its eye teeth (numbers four and five on top) and its stomach teeth (numbers four and five on the bottom). When these teeth come in (at approximately eighteen months), it is the sign of time for weaning, the signal that the child s gastric juices have started to flow. Up to this time the baby needed a pre-digested food, because without gastric juices it could not digest proteins and starches. Cramming cereals and chopped meat into an infant s mouth is stuffing sickness into the baby which will come out later as childhood and adult diseases.

The mother s milk is alkaline, and from this blessed milk (blood transfusion) develops bone, flesh, cartilage, brain and all normal functions of the body. The milk being alkaline is not only accepted, but is for the most part assimilated into the baby s system for good growth. A very small part is not assimilated and is passed off as fecal matter during its bowel movements. This milk is food that has already been digested by the mother, whose gastric juices are doing the work for both of them.

WEANING

When weaning time comes, the child s gastric juices are flowing so it can digest protein and starches on its own. When drinking milk, mother s or cow s, at this time the milk changes from alkaline to acid (being mixed with the gastric juices), and instead of the major part of the milk being assimilated and only a small portion being eliminated, with the gastric juices now altering the picture we have the milk accepted into the body, but only a small part assimilated. The balance is accepted as mucous-forming material that makes for constipation, runny noses, etc.

Stop and think, the only mammals on the face of the earth that will go back to drinking milk after their weaning are a few humans and the household pets around them they have led astray. One farmer I talked to said he has seen an occasional abnormal adult cow suckling on another cow, and he shot the critter without trial.

Dr. William E. Ellis is a retired osteopathic physician and surgeon, located in Arlington, Texas, who has done extensive research on the effects of cow s milk on human beings. His conclusion: Milk and milk products are harmful to many people, both adults and infants. Milk is a contributing factor in constipation, chronic fatigue, arthritis, headaches, muscle cramps, obesity, allergies, and heart problems. Dr . Ellis does not blame cholesterol, but xanthine oxidase (an enzyme in homogenized milk), excess calories, xyramine (a protein in cheese that causes headaches), and poor absorption. He blames especially the latter, as milk neutralizes the hydrochloric acid necessary to digest food and creates excess mucus which inhibits absorption.

Also, allergy to milk is quite common, the symptoms including asthma, nasal congestion, skin rash and various chest infections, plus other less noticed symptoms such as irritability, fatigue, attention deficit disorder (ADD), and hyperactivity. Milk also causes allergies, by diminishing hydrochloric acid necessary to digest protein, causing the undigested protein to enter the bloodstream and promote allergic reactions. The calcium in milk does not metabolize properly, either; Dr. Ellis recommends eating green vegetables, sesame butter and sardines to obtain calcium.

According to historians, one of the greatest days in anyone s life during biblical times was the day of weaning. On that day , the one being honored was the individual that was once a baby, and now that it had cut its eye and stomach teeth was now a child . Family , friends and neighbors were invited to the weaning feast, and who sat at the head of the table? The new child. This is in many instances the only time the individual ever had a special feast of its own with lots of guests, and it was allowed to be honored by sitting at the head of the feasting table.

If the mother of today has been using plenty of the calcium formula and has watched her diet as she should, her baby will be born with a jaw that is full-sized for its age. The upper and lower jaws will develop to the right size to accommodate all thirty-two teeth without crowding them. Crowded teeth result from calcium deficiency, starting with the mother and father (his seed passes on down his weaknesses also.)

Through a proper diet for the parents-to-be and then proper health-giving foods for the child as it matures, there will be no need for tooth braces, wires and misery of this expensive, painful medieval procedure.

With proper diet we have other blessings to pass on to coming generations; namely, a strong, well-built body with adequate calcium to support strong bones, flesh, cartilage, nerves, brain, etc. No need for knock-kneed, bow-legged, polio-infected, weak children with curvature of the spine. We are now going to discuss various diseases and the natural ways to remedy them.

CHAPTER TWO

Treating Illnesses in Children

The pride of having healthy and intelligent children can be the joy of our lives. Through the proper teaching and feeding of our children, and through proper care during illness, we can help raise our children to their highest potential as well as have ease of mind and a peaceful posterity for ourselves.

The advertising media have now convinced the majority of people here on earth that highly refined foods, man-made pharmaceutical drugs, chemotherapy, hormone replacement therapy, x-ray, surgery and relieving the effect instead of clearing the cause of disease are the only way to go. We who believe in the wholistic method of healing mankind are of a far different opinion. This procedure of natural healing has been used with success since the beginning of time.

We believe in using any food, herbal aid, and every kind of therapy that will do good for the body and leave no side- or after-effect. Wholistic foods are wholesome (not processed) and are of a mucusless nature. The word mucus is a confusing term, as people know we have a mucus membrane and we require mucus for our body to work properly. All other mammals of the lower kingdoms need mucus as well. They do not get it from macaroni and cheese, but from fruits, vegetables, grains, nuts and seeds. We can do the same. However, the mucus many of us have in our bodies is a type that is of a dead, low-vibrating substance that cannot be eliminated with ease. This accumulates, layer upon layer, like one layer of wallpaper glued onto another. The dead, inorganic mucus is glue or paste stemming from the materials we take into our bodies under the false terminology of food.

Mucus is the cause of over ninety percent of all diseases. We must choose foods that are free of the harmful mucus and see that the substance we take into our bodies has life in it, not dead foodstuffs that bring on death. Further on in this book we wish to show a wonderful mucusless routine that, if followed, will give a healthy existence to you and yours with an active happy life as long as you want to stay around. Let s clear up the present plague of disease and then start on a new life to keep health from here on out.

In the wholistic program we stress the proper use of herbs. The scriptures say that herbs are to be used with prudence and skill, and all herbs to be used in their wholesome state. In Webster s unabridged dictionary, the word wholesome is defined as: Healthy , whole, entireness; totality; completeness; with the life therein, as in its original state. This rules out processing and man s interference with food s original wholesomeness by altering it to excite the taste buds.

All fruits, vegetables, grains, nuts and seeds are technically herbs. Some are used nutritionally while some, as Ezekiel says, are for medicine. Whether we use them for food or medicine, we do not believe in processing and we do not use poisonous, toxic or habit-forming herbs. We have taught for many years that there are no incurable diseases. Herein is my belief in the wholistic approach as given in one of my newsletters.

THE WHOLISTIC APPROACH

The Wholistic Program of Healing includes procedures that will restore and revitalize any part of the human body. There are several causes for physical malfunctions. Often malnutrition leads to cell deterioration or accidents may cause direct bodily damage. Once an organ or other area of the body is surgically removed, even the wholistic approach to healing is thwarted. At that point only a miracle would restore the body. In the School of Natural Healing, we teach that the body may be renewed when we treat the cause of malfunction and not simply alleviate its effects.

Traditional Judeo-Christian precepts tell us that Deity alone knows what our span of living will be. There is in other words a time to be born and a time to die. Ascribing to these principles it seems illogical that any person would attempt to prescribe for another the term of his living and yet how many times in our years of helping people has a tearful, anguished person come to us having had the end of his or her life foretold by their practitioner? In so many instances we have watched these individuals heal themselves using the recommended wholistic procedures and long outlive their predicted demise.

Of course, as we have often pointed out in our lectures, the rules of wholistic healing may be followed faithfully or they may be followed religiously. The faithful person will adhere strictly to the program of healing, remembering to follow directions as they are given. In the second instance, the ill person treats the principles of wholistic healing the way many of us are religious; that is, we worship only at Christmas or Easter, etc., neglecting the full benefit of faithful adherence.

In the wholistic program only wholesome organic substances are introduced into or applied to the body. They must not be toxic or narcotic and all therapy is for the building up of the body, never damaging its cells. As we have mentioned, the prime purpose of the wholistic program is to restore and revitalize damaged, abnormally functioning organs or body area. Obviously the program is directed towards those who want to enjoy good health and not to the few who enjoy ill health. If you wish to be among those who enjoy and thrive with a healthy body, you will welcome this program and all of its principles of correct, healthful living and thinking.

It is alarming to hear a mother say, When my child was breaking out with chicken pox [measles, or some other childhood disease], he was given some suppressive medication, and only two or three small spots broke out on his body. Here, unknowingly, the parents have gone against nature s procedure for cleaning the toxins out of the body. They have locked in the harmful condition, which may give the body trouble, even many years later.

Many people panic when a child or family member becomes even slightly ill. They rush immediately to any doctor for his advice, shots, pills and the resultant peace of mind from doing what they have been trained to do since childhood to rely on others. In 1969, Utah passed a law stating, in substance, that if a person examines another person with or without charge, they are practicing medicine. It is written that, technically, if a mother says to her child, Y ou have a fever, so I will give you something to help you get better, she is theoretically practicing medicine without a license, and could be arrested on a felony charge. On the other side of the coin there is a statement in this same law that is usually ignored, which reads (again, in substance) that it is permissible to prescribe herbs or old-fashioned household remedies.

DISTILLED WATER DURING ILLNESS

Each day a child should drink an abundance of steam distilled water. This should amount to one ounce of water to each pound of body weight (a thirty-two pound child, one quart or thirty-two ounces). This should not all be used at one time, but distributed throughout the day, as one half in a.m. and the other half p.m.

Distilled water flushes the minerals and inorganic salts that cause sickness out of the body, where juice and other liquids are not as efficient.

There are two types of minerals in the body live organic minerals that can be assimilated into cell structure, and low-vibrating inorganic minerals that are only accepted into the body and cannot be assimilated. These inorganic minerals cause kidney stones, gall stones, hardening of the arteries, poor eyesight, arthritis, etc. People so often say, But why shouldn t I use tap, well, spring, artesian or some other types of hard water to provide minerals for my body? This mineral can be accepted into the body but not assimilated because the hard inorganic minerals must go through plant life and are changed by osmosis to live organic mineral which can then be assimilated into the human cell structure.

We get all the minerals from the fruits, vegetables, grains, nuts and seeds in a form that can all be readily assimilated. The minerals from water and the inorganic, pharmaceutical types can, for the most part, only be accepted but not wholly assimilated. This accumulation of inassimilable minerals can cause side-effects and after-effects.

Distilled water will back out these inorganic minerals, flushing them out of the body, but will not touch or bother the live organic minerals from herb and plant life that the body has assimilated.

We are made from the dust of the earth: From dust thou art, to dust shalt thou return. The minerals in this dust are essential to our bodies so we must acquire from Mother Earth the proper materials to keep the temple of God (our body) in good repair . This is why the following statement from the Old Testament is given us to show us how to get our mineral foods from the dust of Mother Earth. It is Psalms 104:14, which reads: He causeth the grass to grow for the cattle, and herb for the service of man: that he may bring forth food out of the earth. Isn t that a beautifully planned program designed for us?

JUICES

In addition to distilled water, one should drink plenty of juices, freshly-made, if possible, otherwise unsweetened bottled juices will do. Fresh juice is a good food for organic minerals and salts from the earth that can be assimilated to build the body. Of course the body still requires whole foods for roughage and bulk.

HOW TO USE THIS BOOK

Most illnesses have a common cause constipation. This often results in common symptoms, fever and skin eruptions. A brief discussion of these prevalent aspects of illness follows an alphabetized series of specific treatments for diseases, their symptoms and causes, herbs to use for them and how to prepare them. A discussion of the cleansing program and the mucusless diet follow in the appendices, and at the close of the book you will find a list of herbal formulas and other pertinent information you will need in bringing your body back to good health.

In this booklet we have only touched on a few of the aids that can be used to assist people in having a healthier, more optimistic and peaceful outlook on life. For additional reading, see the bibliography.

NOTE: If a condition has progressed to a serious stage, or if uncertainty exists as to the seriousness, it is best not to delay in obtaining the timely professional services of a qualified health care provider.

CHAPTER THREE

Diseases (Listed Alphabetically)

ABSCESS

Definition:

A localized collection of pus (infection) in any part of the body.

Symptoms:

In an abscess we distinguish between the body or center and the sides or edges. The secretions are of different kinds, and upon them depend the benign or malignant character of the abscess. The discharge may consist of one or more of the following: a thin, watery or thick, slimy, clammy, white, green, yellowish green, yellow or bloody, variegated, foul, offensive matter. Benign abscesses heal when the discharge ceases, the cavity or center and side close, and are covered with new skin, although a scar is generally left. A malignant abscess, on the contrary, gives no sign of healing, but rather inclines to get worse, and, if aggravated, to mortify.

Causes:

The causes lie either in local injuries or in a defective blending of blood and other bodily fluids, but generally both circumstances unite in the development of an abscess.

The basic cause of all abscesses, tumors, cysts, etc., stems back to an impure bloodstream which has been fouled by improper food intake which causes poor action of liver and bowels, a faulty digestion, or disturbances in the lymphatic glands. This is generally responsible for the excess accumulation of impurities in the blood.

Herbal Aids:

Apply a poultice over the abscess area of three parts slippery elm bark and one part lobelia herb. A poultice of hops or a poultice of hot onions, hot pumpkin, or hot (not cooked) tomatoes is equally effective. After the abscess has burst, cover it with a poultice or fomentation of comfrey leaves or roots (powdered, or if fresh, finely chopped) for fast healing.

Another useful herbal formula is X-Ceptic which has anti-fungal, anti-bacterial, and antiseptic properties. Apply X-Ceptic to a cotton ball and bandage it over an abscess. This therapy works for infected and abscessed teeth also. Just soak half of a cotton ball in X-Ceptic and place it between the cheek and the infected gums. This fomentation should be changed often and kept on the infection for several hours a day.

One of the best blood-purifying teas is burdock root. Others are chaparral, also known as creosote bush, Oregon grape root, and red clover blossoms. These herbs are found in the Blood Stream Formula (Red Clover Combination)

Dosage: Be generous in making poultices, covering the afflicted areas very thickly. As an abscess ripens it will get larger and continue to expand until it bursts open and drains. After the pus and solid matters are nearly drained off, fluid, sometimes bloody, will run from the abscess. This is when you put on the comfrey poultice or fomentation.

ACIDOSIS

Definition:

Excessive acidity of the body fluids due to an accumulation of acids or an excessive reduction of alkali reserves, due to an excess of acid-forming foods which are incompletely oxidized or poorly eliminated. This leads to the cause of stomach disorders. As Otto Mausert, N.D., states in his book *Herbs*, the body needs sodium (bicarbonate), potassium, calcium, and magnesium. Acidosis is the depletion of these alkali reserves.

Symptoms:

Loss of appetite, headaches, sleeplessness, acidic urine, acidic or strong perspiration, acid mouth, sour stomach, and vomiting.

Causes:

As Otto Mausert states:

Stomach disorders There are different diseases caused by acidosis coming under this heading, but the direct cause is the same for almost all of them. Eating fast, improper chewing, overloading, and eating the wrong kinds of food, are generally responsible for the troubles. The bad habits must be abandoned in order to affect a cure, as there is no medicine that can chew the food properly, or stop anybody from overloading, or prevent one from eating things that are hard to digest.

Food that is not properly masticated is retained longer in the stomach than it should be. As a result, it turns sour and ferments, creating an excessive amount of acid and gas. This in turn causes a great deal of irritation and inflammation on the mucus lining of the whole digestive system or tract. A catarrhal condition gradually sets in, and the lining becomes coated with a thick slimy mucus that interferes with the assimilation of the food. Decomposition and decay result. Poisonous matter therefrom is absorbed, which leads to severe disturbances of the stomach and bowels and gradually the whole system. The result of this is far reaching, as it finally leads to many other diseases to which the human race is heir. It is only too true, that most people dig their own graves with their teeth.

Let me therefore repeat, what we might call the Golden Rule of Health: eat slowly, chew food well, and don t overload. Eat only plain food, plenty of fresh vegetable matter, salads, ripe fruits. The richer foods, however, such as meat, eggs, starches, sweets, etc., should be taken more moderately and only in proportion to the amount of work one does. In that way the food can be balanced properly and digested more completely. Failure to live up to these simple natural rules will gradually lead to the operating table but the operation will not remove the underlying cause, and consequently will not bring the desired relief.

We have another author who is a wise old doctor of the past, who gives his view as follows (Jethro Kloss in Back to Eden):

> Acidosis Causes Meats, fish, fowl, tea, coffee, tobacco, alcohol, pepper (cooked), mustard, spices, vinegar, excessive uses of salt, baking powder, soda, jellies, sweet desserts (not the natural sweets), candy, preserves, pancakes, hot breads, pastries, fried foods, irregular eating, eating late at night, excess starch, improperly cooked foods, starchy and poorly baked bread, foods too hot or too cold, and foods cooked in aluminum utensils.

Herbal Aids:

Aids to soothe and speed up the healing are slippery elm gruel, marshmallow root tea, okra, carrot and spinach juice. Peppermint tea is also an excellent beverage for this condition. To assist it in its stimulating effect, add six to ten drops of tincture of lobelia, or antispasmodic tincture to each cup of tea. The use of potassium broth is a great aid; spinach juice, mixed with carrot juice, is also excellent.

Treatment:

Use the instructions for Dr. Christopher s Three-Day Cleansing Program and Mucusless Diet described in Appendix B. If the condition is severe, follow instructions for the Incurables, found in Appendix D. Keep the bowels clean and the eliminative channels moving freely, as outlined in Appendix A.

The food should be eaten as dry as possible, mixing thoroughly with saliva to a liquid form, not drinking liquids with the meals. The drier the food is eaten, the sooner the acid condition can be overcome. Chew! Chew! Chew! so that your food is liquefied before swallowing.

Sodium and magnesium foods such as oranges (whole, not the juice), beets, carrots, celery, cucumbers, okra, radishes, apples, cherries, strawberries, coconuts, figs, prunes, string beans, and spinach, should be eaten in abundance.

ACNE AND SKIN PROBLEMS

Definition:

Acne is a chronic inflammatory condition affecting skin structures usually involving the face, back and chest. It usually affects those between the age of puberty and the twenties.

Symptoms:

The primary lesion or blackhead develops into a pinkish pustule or nodule. A teenager, sometime preteen, often breaks out with a horrible skin condition in which pustules and their scars may cover the skin, which is often coarse and oily. This may cause an inferiority complex and other emotional disruption. At this time they may become irritable, snap and snarl at people. They seem impossible to be around why? They are growing into adulthood so rapidly that they are maturing faster than they are equipped.

Causes:

As the teenagers grow up, they, like everybody else today, eat devitalized, dead, mucus-loaded junk materials that could only be called garbage food, and meals without energy and life building materials in them. The rapid change from childhood to adulthood requires foods rich in vitamins, minerals, etc., needed in the healthy body. Processed foods are low or lacking in natural hormone and estrogen materials needed in the growth transition to adulthood. The young person s body realizes the lack and the need, and tries to pull the required materials from the body. If they are not there, the strain of trying to produce them causes irritation, a nasty emotional disposition, and a pimply complexion.

We blame the child for not being cooperative, for craving sweets, excess meats and bakery products. The body is craving vitamins and minerals and basic needs for health, and that craving is termed hidden hunger. To pacify this hungry gnawing feeling, the young person stuffs on junk food, adding insult to injury. From this diet comes acne, boils, irritability, and a sick, sad youth. The girls have difficult menstrual periods with cramps, flooding, or off-timed cycles, and the boys have a tendency toward early prostrate trouble and unhealthy sex drive.

Herbal Aids:

During puberty, and preferably just before that time starts, it would be wise to have the preteen boy and girl take a cup or more of red raspberry leaf tea and/or (especially important) blessed (holy) thistle tea each day six days each week. These teas will assist in supplying natural hormone and estrogen materials to the system. As a side note, puberty is also much easier to go through if the tonsils are still intact (see tonsillitis). The condition of the skin is often a reflection of the condition of the liver. For this reason, we have seen much success when using the Liver Gall Bladder Formula (Barberry LG).

Other Treatments:

We often wonder how we can control the cravings of our youth for junk foods with all the pizza parlors, hamburger stands and malt-shops open. It is easier to educate the children early, by teaching them to acquire the habit of eating and wanting good wholesome food, instead of developing these cravings. The body, or temple, is then clean and when they have good satisfying foods at home it is much easier to live with all the junk foods in the world and ignore them! We have watched parents rear their children on the mucusless diet using plenty of fruits, vegetables, grains, nuts and seeds. These children went into adulthood and through the puberty stage with flying colors no acne, and with a sweet, pleasing disposition.

ADENOIDS-SWELLING

Definition:

The adenoids are two swellings at the back of the nose, just above the tonsils. They are made up of lymph nodes which form part of the body s defense against upper respiratory tract infections.

Causes:

In most children, adenoids shrink after the age of about five years, disappearing altogether by puberty. In some children, however, they become even larger and obstruct the passage from the nose to the throat, causing snoring, breathing through the mouth, and a characteristically nasal voice. They can also block the eustachian tubes (which connects the middle ear to the throat), causing infection and deafness. (Taken from The Medical Association Encyclopedia of Medicine, Random House)

The polyps are caused by a toxic and mucus condition in the body, so go back to the basic cause and use the mucusless diet (see Appendix B).

Herbal Aids:

To shrink the swellings in the nose and throat areas, make a tea of bayberry bark or oak bark and sniff it up the nose. Children can be taught to drink it up the nose using one nostril at a time. It will also be helpful to drink some of this tea two or three times a day. For some, the easier way is to use an atomizer spray up the nose. Still another procedure is to put a pinch of the oak bark or bayberry bark powder into a plastic, flexible drinking straw, and, very carefully, blow it up the nose (only a very small amount at a time or it will plug up the nose and get into the lungs).

Other Treatment:

The regular use of fresh carrot juice is a fine aid to clean up the mucus membrane and reduce the unnatural swellings in the body including the adenoids.

ALLERGIES

Definition:

Physical discomfort, irritation or reaction to specific substances which normally would not cause hypersensitivity in the body.

Symptoms:

The patient may sneeze and cough, suffer from a runny nose and excess mucus, and have swollen or irritated eyes. The skin may erupt in rashes, and there may be a headache or sore throat, as in a common cold. In extreme cases the sufferer may go into anaphylactic shock which is life-threatening.

Causes:

The immune system is exposed to foreign protein either through blood exchange in the digestive tract, vaccination, etc. The immune system develops a sensitivity to this protein and reacts as though it was being invaded. This reaction is called an allergy.

Dr. Harold Thomas Hyman, M.D., in his book *Handbook of Differential Diagnosis* (Philadelphia, London, Montreal: J.B. Lippincott Co.) explains that despite limitations in current understanding of the problem, the state of allergy is described best as a perversion or perversions of the mechanisms of host-defense. Several pages then continue to explain whether the allergies are histamine versus tuberculin type and the many tests, clinically, to determine the cause. The cause can be pollen, plants, micro-organisms and their products, animal tissues, digestants, cosmetics, drugs, serums, articles of clothing, dyes, industrial products, physical modalities (heat, cold, solar energy, etc.), and psychic tensions. The first step in cleaning up the cause of allergies is to work on rebuilding the bowel area to a healthy cleansing action (see Appendix A).

Herbal Aids:

Clean the blood stream with a good herbal tea such as the Blood Stream Formula (Red Clover Combination), which consists of red clover blossoms, chaparral, licorice root, poke root, peach bark, Oregon grape root, stillingia, prickly ash bark, burdock root, and buckthorn bark. A very fine herbal remedy for allergies, hay fever and sinus conditions is the Sinus Plus Formula (SHA Tea) which consists of: Brigham tea, marshmallow root, juniper berries, goldenseal root, chaparral, burdock root, parsley root, cayenne, lobelia. Adult dose:

one cup morning and evening. We have had a lot of success using the Immucalm Formula for all types of allergies including auto-immune disorders (when the immune system is attacking the body itself) including arthritis, multiple sclerosis, Type 1 Diabetes etc. Another aid for sinus-stopped-up head and nose is our horseradish combination, described below.

Preparation:

Blend fresh, chopped-up horseradish roots into apple cider vinegar making a thick pulp. Chew one-fourth teaspoonful of the pulp thoroughly before swallowing, and do this three times during a day. Each three days increase this amount by one-eighth teaspoon until one teaspoonful is being taken.

Other Treatment:

Use the three-day cleanse once every thirty days, or at least once every three months and follow the mucusless diet. (See Appendix B.)

Be sure to drink at least one gallon of distilled water per day for an adult of average size. We use one ounce of distilled water to each pound of weight per day twenty ounces for a twenty pound child. One who weighs one-hundred and thirty pounds would use one-hundred and thirty ounces per day, or about one gallon.

ANEMIA

Definition:

Anemia is a deficiency in the number of red blood cells, hemoglobin or both.

Symptoms:

The condition is marked by varying degrees of pallor and palpitation.

Causes:

When we have a good bloodstream we have a good, healthy

life. It would be wise to take time to learn the principles of building good blood in the body. One of our teachers, Dr. Edward E. Shook at the Los Angeles Herbal Institute, gives a fine explanation of the cause of anemia as follows:

> Carbon dioxide and other waste gasses are reabsorbed into the life-giving oxygen. Everyone knows that two atoms of oxygen unite with one atom of carbon to form dioxide. But when there is insufficient oxygen, only one atom unites with carbon, to produce carbon-monoxide, and that is where most of our trouble begins anemia, low blood pressure, or where there is an abundance of calcium, high blood pressure; because calcium thickens the blood. It requires a great deal more pressure to pump thick blood than it does to pump thin blood; and please make special note, that all this is brought about because there is not sufficient iron in the blood, to carry enough oxygen to the cells, to enable them to breathe, and throw off their waste products. New cells are not produced fast enough to replace the decaying and dead ones. Pus is formed only when cells decay. Therefore, it requires no great stretch of the imagination to see how vitally necessary it is to have enough iron in the blood stream to convey sufficient oxygen to all parts.
>
> Nearly every food we eat, or a large percentage of it, contains iron and oxygen. Wheat and most of the grains and cereals (in their whole state) contain iron in the form of iron phosphate, as do many vegetables, such as beets, turnips, tomatoes, spinach, lettuce, cabbage, celery, carrots, squash, parsley, mustard greens, dandelion leaves, watercress, etc., but our principal source of organic iron and oxygen is the fruit. The apple is loaded with these two elements, particularly the winesap. All berries, plums, prunes, grapes, raisins, dates, figs, cherries, etc., contain organic iron in abundance, and the citrus fruits, such as oranges, lemons, limes, etc., are principally composed of citric acid, which is one third oxygen.

Herbal Aids:

Here is an excellent herbal tea for delicate and weak children with pale and sallow skin, anemia, and general malnutrition. This is a superb remedy and is perfectly harmless, and therefore can be taken in large doses, but should not be given to a point of causing diarrhea. This remedy will keep for a long time if kept in a cool place and well corked:

4 ounces of barberry bark (cut)
3 pints of distilled water

Put the bark into the water and let it stand one hour. Simmer slowly until the water barely covers the herb. Strain through a cloth and set this liquid aside. Return the herb to the saucepan and cover with one quart of water. Simmer again for fifteen to twenty minutes. Strain and add the two liquids together. Put into a clean saucepan and slowly reduce by simmering to one pint. Take from the heat and add eight fluid ounces of vegetable glycerine. Cool and bottle. Dose: One teaspoonful to a tablespoonful three times a day. Children: a half to one teaspoonful in honey water three times a day until the bowels are acting freely, then reduce the dose.

Another great aid in anemia is comfrey. This herb can be used in the form of comfrey tea, tablets, capsules, in salads and in comfrey green drink. Make the green drink by blending into apple juice (or some pleasant-tasting vegetable juice, such as fresh carrot), comfrey, marshmallow root, parsley, spinach, and other greens (Jurassic Green Powder may also be used). Sweeten with honey and use a cup morning and night (a half cup for children). Each mouthful of the juice should be chewed thoroughly (swished in the mouth) and mixed well with saliva before swallowing. The use of grapes, grape juice and raisins in an abundance is excellent in rebuilding an iron-deficient bloodstream.

Another of our fine tonics follows:

2 ounces yellow dock root powder
4 ounces sarsaparilla root powder
2 ounces comfrey root powder

1/2 ounce sassafras bark powder

Simmer the above ingredients in two quarts of water and reduce to one quart; strain, dissolve sufficient honey to make into a syrup, allow to cool, bottle and keep in a cool place. Two teaspoonfuls to one tablespoonful after each meal.

These are wonderful aids and suggestions to rebuild the blood stream to perfection, but be sure to always go back to the cause and keep the bowels clean.

Other Treatments:

Whenever the child or adult has anemia, which is a deficiency of blood in quantity as well as quality, the overall treatment should be sunshine, fresh air, deep breathing, and a well balanced diet including a healthy quantity of fresh, green vegetables and the daily use of good tonic herbal supplements.

APPENDICITIS

Definition:

Appendicitis is inflammation of the appendix, sometimes resulting in rupture.

Symptoms:

The symptoms of appendicitis are an inflamed, painful condition of the appendix and the surrounding portion of the bowels. Other symptoms are nausea, pain and distress around the navel, constipation, quick pulse, and perhaps a rise in temperature to 100 or 102 degrees F. There may be tenderness to the right of the navel and below, which is increased by pressure or movement. The patient frequently flexes the right knee to ease the pain.

Causes:

It may be caused by a faulty digestion, intestinal catarrh, fecal concretions and, in comparatively rare cases, by foreign particles being lodged in the appendix. This is the explanation given by Otto Mausert, N.D., *Herbs* (Elaine M. Muhr).

Dr. Kloss states:

> Constipation is one of the causes of appendicitis to an extent, and of course, wrong diet, which diet would include the use of devitalized foods such as white flour products, cane sugar, and cane sugar products (all refined sugars), greasy and fried foods, tea, coffee, chocolate, and wrong combinations of foods. These must be strictly avoided in appendicitis, as must alcoholic drinks, tobacco, and all stimulating food and drink .

Treatment:

Dr. Kloss recommends:

> Cleanse the colon thoroughly with an enema, preferably herb, take as much water as possible, as hot as possible. The treatment is of great value and will often relieve the pain immediately. If using an herb enema, use either spearmint, catnip, white oak bark, bayberry or wild alum root. When herbs are not available, use plain water. If the pain continues after the colon has been cleansed, then use a very warm enema of catnip alone. Then apply hot and cold fomentations to the region of the appendix and the full length of the spine. This will aid in the cleaning process and relieve pain. At night prepare a poultice as follows: Combine a tablespoon of granulated or powdered lobelia with a large handful of granulated or crushed mullein leaves, and sprinkle with ginger. Mix the herbs into a paste by adding powdered slippery elm or corn meal. Apply the poultice as warm as the patient can stand, leave on cool, then repeat. When suffering an attack of appendicitis, go on a liquid diet, drinking alkaline broths, fruit juices, and drink several glasses of slippery elm (or comfrey) every day. Traditional Chinese medicine advocates Chinese Rhubarb (a mild laxative) and lightly stroking the painful area. Alternating hot and cold castor oil fomentations brings tremendous relief.

See also *Dr. Christopher s Guide to Colon Health* for the

complete herbal protocol for Appendicitis. After an individual is over an attack (which is the effect), go immediately onto the mucusless diet as suggested by Dr. Christopher (see Appendix B).

ASTHMA

Definition:

Asthma is a chronic respiratory disease which affects the bronchial tubes.

Symptoms:

It is often called allergic asthma, characterized by dyspnea (labored breathing), cough, wheezing, mucoid sputum, bronchial spasm, and a sense of constriction of the chest. The system is filled with waste matter and mucus. Asthma is characterized by a dry and painful cough which is often due to an extreme irritation of the mucous membranes in the nasal passages or bronchial tubes. The symptoms are accompanied by constriction of the chest (bronchiolar spasm) and expectoration of mucus (mucoid sputum). Asthma may result in an excessive development (hypertrophy) of the glandular elements. This affliction is commonly believed to be due to hypersensitivity to inhaled or ingested substances such as odors, pollen, dust, smoke, etc.

Causes:

Asthma is caused by malnutrition. Only by diligent and consistent effort to change embedded habits will one get permanent relief. The cough is a result of nature s effort to expectorate mucus from the lungs, after which breathing becomes easier. Often the cause of asthma is basically a nervous condition because the nerves are irritated.

Herbal Aids:

When a person is in convulsion there are certain herbs that will give very fast relief. One of these is tincture of lobelia, and a valerian decoction with a little cayenne added to relieve spasms. If such an attack comes after a meal, one should use an emetic, such as a large dose of lobelia or use the yoga finger method. Drink several cups of warm water, then place the middle finger deep down the throat and press the tongue until regurgitation starts. Mustard is also good to clean the stomach and lungs.

Prior to the emetic, a peppermint, cayenne, or spearmint tea should be used as a stimulant to soothe the area and alleviate the discomfort of continual vomiting. Hot fomentations of castor oil, comfrey, lobelia and mullein, may be placed over the stomach, spleen, liver and lung areas. Frequent hydrotherapy baths or lengthy sweat baths are beneficial, followed by a cold shower or sponging. Another helpful method is to take a vapor bath twice a week, inhaling steam from a decoction of ragwort or wormwood. A decoction of equal parts of the following herbs, taken warm will prove very beneficial: elecampane root, horehound, hyssop, skunk cabbage root, vervain, wild cherry bark (and to this preparation add a few drops of tincture of lobelia or Antispasmodic tincture). Clear the bowels with an injection of catnip or barberry bark. This affliction also calls for plenty of outdoor exercise, deep breathing, and good ventilation while sleeping. The whole body system should be strengthened with tonic herbs such as chickweed, comfrey, marshmallow, and mullein. The diet should be mostly fruits and vegetables, avoiding all processed and devitalized (dead) foods.

The following formulas are two excellent aids for nourishing and giving ease to asthma:

Lung and Bronchial Formula (Resp-Free): This combination of herbs is an aid to relieve irritation in the respiratory tract lungs and bronchials. This is an aid in emphysema as well as other bronchial and lung congestion such as bronchitis, asthma, tuberculosis, etc. Suggested amount of these would be two or three times in a day. Additional aid is sometimes received by taking this combination with a cup of comfrey tea. The ingredients of the respiratory combination are marshmallow, mullein, comfrey, lobelia, and chickweed, in equal parts.

Sinus Plus Formula (SHA-Tea): This combination is a natural herbal aid working as a decongestant and antihistamine to dry up sinuses and expel from the head and bronchopulmonary tubes and

passages the offending stoppage and mucus. Combine this with the Lung and Bronchial Formula to speed up the process. The ingredients of this formulas are Brigham tea, marshmallow, goldenseal root, chaparral, burdock root, parsley, lobelia and cayenne.
Additional Treatment:

Asthma sufferers will greatly speed up their healing process by immediately stopping use of all dairy products, white flour and refined sugars, as these products contribute to harmful, excess mucus in the system.

As stated before, asthma results from malnutrition, and even though the patient has recovered with the procedures mentioned herein, the wise person will turn to fresh, wholesome foods and beverages to keep the body in a perfect state. This will guarantee permanent relief by removing the cause of dis-ease.

BED WETTING

Definition:

Bed wetting is the inability to withhold urine during sleep.

Symptoms:

Aside from the obvious difficulty, the child is often nervous and may suffer from digestion troubles. At times it is difficult for children and adults to control voiding of urine. They urinate unconsciously, wet the bed, or cannot get to the restroom quickly enough. Ads in the magazines recommend special guards pads and diapers to wear during the day for these youths and adults. This is working on the effect! Let s get to the cause. This condition of incontinence or enuresis (involuntary flowing of urine) can be helped by feeding the malfunction organs; namely the kidneys, bladder, and urethral tubes, with herbal foods rich in the elements missing for a good healthy body and organs of elimination.

Cause:

Bed wetting or incontinence of urine is frequently due to the presence of inorganic oxalic acid crystals in the kidneys or bladder.

This disagreeable trouble is due to an involuntary relaxation and weakness of the muscle that closes the bladder. This is also known as enuresis, caused by wrong diet. Weak and undernourished children with a lack of wholesome food are most likely to have this habit. Other causes are late suppers, constipation, worms, gas in bowels, and general nervousness. Do not scold or spank the child for bed wetting, as this causes the child to become more nervous because of the scoldings and punishments. Why not try to kindly remonstrate and then help them as we will explain, by going to the cause. This embarrassing habit is one any child dislikes, but needs help from the parents to overcome.

Herbal Aids

The Kidney Formula (Juni-Pars) is used as an aid of kidney it is made from the following herbs: Juniper berries, parsley, uva ursi, marshmallow root, lobelia, ginger, and goldenseal. Suggested use is two or more capsules morning and evening with a cup of parsley tea.

One of the finest herbal combinations for bed-wetting, which we have used for many years is the Bladder Formula (DRI or Kid-e-Dry) it contains: marshmallow root, black cohosh, parsley root, uva ursi, juniper berries, white pond lily, goldenseal, ginger, white poplar, sumach berries, yarrow. Use these in powder form, place in number two capsule, and give two or more morning and evening with parsley tea. If the child cannot swallow capsules, take the powder and mix with honey or blackstrap molasses (the Kid-e-Dry formula is in a sweet liquid base (glycerine), made for children that have a hard time swallowing capsules.)

Make a tea of plantain, black cohosh and parsley root, one half to one fourth cup three times a day. Sweeten with honey, if desired. These herbs may be in powder form if desired and placed into number 0 capsules the dosage is one capsule three times a day.

Thoroughly mix together buchu leaves, marshmallow root, black cohosh, yarrow, uva ursi, white pond lily, juniper berries, goldenseal, and ginger. Put the well-mixed powders into number 0 capsules and give two each night and morning with a cup of parsley tea.

Additional Treatments:

Do not let the child eat late at night or eat any stimulating foods, such as tea, coffee, soft drinks, white flour or white sugar products. It is best to give the child no food or liquids after four or five o clock. Use a gentle olive oil massage daily over the kidney area. The child should not lie on their back; they should lie on their side or face. A good aid for this is to make a large firm cloth ball and fasten into the middle of the back. This can be done by putting the ball onto the back of the night clothes, etc. Make the ball by rolling strips of old cloth or stocking into a ball, stitching it so it will not fall apart. During the night the child starts sleeping on their side, later rolling onto the back. The ball is uncomfortable, so, in sleep, he rolls over to the other side.

Do not give bed-wetters liquids just before retiring, but have them take the last teas or beverages several hours before going to bed. They can always eat ripe fruit for quenching the thirst and this will often give more satisfaction.

BRONCHITIS

Definition:

Bronchitis is the inflammation of the bronchial tubes.

Symptoms:

Acute bronchitis is often accompanied by chills and fever, tightness and stuffiness in the chest, and sometimes a severe cough. In chronic bronchitis, there are almost continual coughing spasms producing quantities of mucus, and shortness of breath.

Causes:

This condition is due to excessive mucus in the system, or

excessive accumulation of retained waste. Constipation is one of the chief causes of the problem. If Nature s warnings are ignored, she will furnish the body with germs and bacteria to do the scavenging of this debris, which can result in influenza or pneumonia (inflammation of the lungs). Relieving the effects of the condition alone will not heal it. You must go to the cause. Bronchitis usually develops from a cold which settles in the lungs and develops into a chronic condition. If not healed, it eventually goes into consumption or tuberculosis. The basic cause, again, is refined, devitalized, processed foods that have lost their original wholesome value.

Herbal Aids:

Comfrey, mullein and lobelia are excellent herbs for relieving bronchitis these can be found in the Lung and Bronchial Formula (Resp Free). The bowel must be cleared (see Appendix A) and kept open with the Lower Bowel Formula, or by adding pre-soaked and low heated flaxseed and/or psyllium seed to whole pre-soaked and low-heated grains (wheat, rye, millet, buckwheat, barley, etc.). If there is a shortness of breath, and an immediate need for the throat to be cleared of mucus, use an emetic such as lobelia or cayenne in a tea of chickweed, marshmallow, and comfrey. One can relax the throat, stomach, and bronchi very rapidly with a few drops of lobelia tincture. Other formulas that are helpful are the Cold Season Formula (GR&P), and the Super Garlic Immune Formula (Anti-Plague.)

Other Treatments:

Healing will be greatly aided by stopping all dairy products, white flour and refined sugar.

Other useful aids for relief are a hot vapor or steam bath followed by a cold shower or sponging; also hot fomentations of pleurisy root and/or mullein (with lobelia in it) on the chest and spine. If you want to speed up any fomentation, add cayenne as a counterirritant.

BURNS AND SUNBURNS

Definition and Causes:

Burns are the result of damage to the skin by some source of heat, such as the sun, fires, stoves, or chemicals.

Symptoms:

A mild burn, often termed first-degree, results in a reddening of the skin. More severe burns, second-degree, may show blisters in addition to the redness, while extremely severe or third-degree burns always show blisters and usually consist of damage to deeper tissue, and present the possibility of scarring.

Herbal Aids:

The following paste formula can be used for the mildest to the most severe third-degree burns with assurance of healing, if used as instructed. This paste has been used by hundreds of people with great success, and is made as follows. To equal parts of liquid honey and wheat germ oil, blend in finely chopped or powdered fresh or dried comfrey leaf or root. When the mixture is the consistency of a heavy spreadable paste, it is ready to use. Apply it a half-inch thick or more over the entire area that has been burned, scalded, etc. Cover with gauze and bandage lightly. Observe the burned area from day to day. If paste has been absorbed, add more on top of the original application. Do not remove original paste application, just add to it when needed. This paste will keep well for many months at room temperature if kept in a tightly closed jar. Always have it on hand for emergencies. You might want to carry a small jar on trips in case of emergency.

Other Treatment:

If the paste is not available, submerge the burned area in cold water and leave it there as long as possible to take the heat out, or keep cold wet compresses over the burned area. If honey, wheat germ oil, or olive oil are available, use them to saturate the area completely, keeping it well soaked in the honey or oil until healed. The gel from the aloe vera plant promotes the healing of burns, and The Complete Tissue

Formula (BF&C) is also quite helpful. These are all good, but nothing can compare to the comfrey paste.

BROKEN BONES

Herbal Aids:

After the doctor has set the bone, drink three or more cups of comfrey tea each day the more the better . With each cup of tea take The Herbal Calcium Formula (Calc-Tea). This is the formula. Which contains horsetail grass, comfrey root, oat straw, and lobelia. Also, use The Complete Tissue Formula (BF&C). This formula comes in ointment, oil, and in capsules. Take between twelve and forty capsules each day and apply the ointment or oil to the affected area several times a day.

For children old enough to take capsules, use two number 00 capsules or more, three times in a day. As suggested, take these capsules with the comfrey tea. Mix the powder with blackstrap molasses, if it is hard to swallow the capsules. Most children prefer the Kid-e-Calc formula which is made with glycerine and tastes sweet.

Additional Treatments:

See the section on tooth care.

CANKER

Definition:

Ulceration, chiefly of the mouth and lips; aphthous stomatitis.

Symptoms:

Painful sores on the inside of the cheeks, lips, etc.

Causes:

Cankers are generally caused by toxicity or over-acidity in the body which does not allow wounds in the mouth to heal. It is a condition not only in the mouth, but all through the entire system.

Herbal Aids:

Keep the patient on juices, distilled water and red raspberry-leaf tea for three days (they will not starve), and you will see the general improvement of the condition. If they want more to eat, give him comfrey green drink, slippery elm bark tea, or marshmallow root tea.

Other Treatment:

The patient should follow the mucusless diet and keep the bowels clean and free moving so that there will be no recurrence.

CARDIAC (HEART) TROUBLE

Definition:

General heart disorder.

Symptoms:

Weakness of the heart, palpitations, etc.

Causes:

Inherent weakness, malnutrition, poor assimilation.

Herbal Aids:

The heart will improve with our program of the mucusless diet (see Appendix B), but to speed up healing it is good to add herbal foods that are specific in rejuvenating and rebuilding the heart area. Two excellent remedies are hawthorn berry and cayenne pepper. It is good for aiding the weak heart to use cayenne each day as explained in The Mucusless Diet supplements in Appendix B.

In case of a sudden heart attack, use a teaspoonful of cayenne in a cup of hot water, and have the patient drink the full cup. Follow with the diet, bowel cleaning and heart foods from then on until healing is fully evident. One of the finest aids is Hawthorn Berry Syrup, an herbal food for the heart. This contains hawthorn berry juice, grape brandy and glycerine. Take 1/4 to 1/2 teaspoon three times a day. To relieve high blood pressure and other circulatory problems, use the Blood Circulation Formula (BPE). This formula contains herbal foods that clean, feed and rebuild the circulatory system.

Additional Treatment:

Another great aid is a tablespoon of wheat germ oil mixed in a comfrey green drink each day. You may also want to try blending powdered comfrey leaves or root (preferably fresh) into pineapple or apple juice, apricot nectar, etc. Add a few dandelion plants and some honey or blackstrap molasses, and to this mixture blend in the wheat germ oil, so it is not oily.

CHICKEN POX

Definition:

Chicken pox is an acute contagious disease of childhood.

Symptoms:

Chicken pox is marked by a slight fever, characterized by superficial eruption of macular transparent vesicles appearing in successive crops on different parts of the body. They rarely become pustular, but dry up, and are only occasionally followed by scars. The duration of the disease is about a week, during which time it usually runs a very mild course. The chicken pox virus propagates in a medium of excess mucus. In the absence of such medium (mucus from excessive starches and sugars, etc.), the virus cannot thrive.

Causes:

Actually, as long as the child has been exposed, the condition is there. A good break-out of chicken pox, as with most childhood diseases, is a blessing. This is the indication that the body has toxic materials in it that must be removed.

Herbal Aids:

Give the child a warm catnip tea enema. Herbal teas such as catnip and peppermint, pleurisy root and catnip, red raspberry leaf, and yarrow or pennyroyal, elder flowers and peppermint with vinegar and water will relieve the itching. Also, bathe or sponge skin with tea made of burdock root, goldenseal and yellow dock root in case of severe itching.

Treatment:

During an outbreak of chicken pox, the body is sending toxic impurities out through the pores. We can aid this by giving the child warm yarrow tea, one cup every hour or two. As a diaphoretic, yarrow opens the pores, causing the body to perspire, and aids in quickly removing the toxins from the system. Itching is generally very mild when this method is used, and the duration of the infection much shorter.

It is also helpful to cleanse the body and to follow a program of moist heat to bring out a good showing of the pox. Use the following instruction for all types of high fever diseases (See Appendix C). If the child is slow in breaking out, give him a good hot bath. Have him drink lots of liquids throughout the day fruit and vegetable juices, lemonade sweetened with honey (no sugars), and fruits. If this program is followed, the disease should follow a mild course with little discomfort.

COLIC

Definition:

Pertaining to the colon: acute abdominal pain or gas pains, often due to improper combination of food and retention of waste matter in the system. Enemas will usually give immediate, but only temporary, relief.

Symptoms:

Paroxysmal abdominal pains due to smooth muscle spasm, obstruction by calculi, nervous indigestion or distention or enlargement of any of the hollow viscera.

Causes:

In all cases, this is due to improper diet, digestive disorder and poor elimination.

Herbal Aids:

A tea or tincture of catnip and fennel is especially helpful for infants. This herbal combination can be found as the Kid-e-Col formula in a base of glycerine. As an infusion, a pint of boiling distilled water over a handful of fresh parsley is also good.

A good formula for children s colic is equal parts of wild yam, pleurisy root, cinnamon and anise. Mix and use one teaspoon of the combined herbs to a cup of boiling water, cover and steep for twenty minutes, strain and add honey, and give dose of one or two tablespoons of tea each fifteen minutes or as needed.

Use the Composition Powder as follows: four parts bayberry bark powder, two parts ginger powder, one part pinus or hemlock spruce inner bark powder, one eighth part clove powder, and one eighth part cayenne powder.

Preparation:

Mix and strain through a fine sieve at least twice. Use one teaspoon in one cupful of boiling water, sweeten, cover and allow to stand a few minutes. Dosage: drink the clear liquid as needed according to age. For example, only part of a teaspoon every hour or two for a very small child.

Additional Treatments:

In addition to taking teas orally, give a rectal injection of teas, two ounces at a time, of catnip, catnip and pleurisy root, garden sage and catnip, or catnip and peppermint. It is an advantage to add three to ten drops of tincture of lobelia to the teas per cup and one-half teaspoon or more of the tincture of lobelia to the rectal injection or massaged over the abdomen.

COLDS, CATARRH, CORYZA, INFLUENZA

Definition:

A cold is a disorder in the respiratory tract resulting from exposure, with catarrh and invasion of microbial cleansers.

Symptoms:

Common cold, coryza, cold in the head, etc. are evidenced by an inflammation of the upper respiratory tract, marked by an acute catarrhal condition of the nasal mucous membrane, a slight rise in the temperature, chilly sensations and general discomfort.

Causes:

It is caused by viral or bacterial infection feeding on excessive or copious secretions of mucus (waste materials) often due to the body s inability to properly assimilate milk and concentrated starches. When a cold or fever just gets started, it can be cleared up very easily, if the following procedures are started immediately.

Herbal Aids:

One of the most simple remedies is to stop the use of all foods and beverages, take a high herbal enema (catnip is good), and drink only red raspberry leaf tea. Between cups of this tea, distilled water may be used, and, if desired, give the patient some good organic vitamin C. Some excellent sources are oranges and fresh orange juice, rose hips, and cayenne. It is possible to use quarts of red raspberry tea during the day and nothing else. For children, use according to age. The runny nose, fever, headache and weariness will leave and they will feel like a new person. Even after feeling greatly improved, continue with the red raspberry leaf tea all that day and well into the next day. If an adult would stay on the tea for three days it would do a wonderful cleaning job for the body.

Preparation:

To make red raspberry leaf tea use one heaping teaspoonful of cut or powdered raspberry leaves into a teacup. Fill the cup with boiling distilled water, cover and let stand in a warm place for five or ten minutes. Strain, and drink it while it is very warm.

Both raspberry leaves and berries contain a very wonderful citrate of iron. It is upon these God-given formulas that the body depends for the remarkable blood-making and regulating properties (astringent and contracting action on internal tissues and membranes). The leaves also contain pectin and other organic acids, calcium and potassium chloride and sulphate. Medicinal action and uses of raspberry leaf tea are astringent, tonic, hemostatic, antiseptic, anti-abortifacient, parturient, anti-gonorrheal, anti-leucorrheal and anti-malarial. With this description of a simple herbal tea, can you now doubt why it is so good for mankind? In Ezekiel we are told 47:12 and the fruit thereof shall be for meat, and the leaf thereof for medicine.

Another simple procedure is when you feel a cold or flu coming on in the evening, use boneset tea. This herb is a nervine stimulant, tonic, diaphoretic, diuretic, and in large doses, emetic, aperient. This is a wonderful remedy for breaking a chill in intermittent fever, muscular rheumatism, bronchitis, influenza, dyspepsia, sore throat, etc.

To use boneset tea, take one ounce of cut boneset herb and over it pour 1 1/4 pints of boiling distilled water. Cover and set in a hot place to steep (do not boil) for thirty minutes.

As one of our favorite teachers, Dr. Shook, expressed it:

> In our long experience with herbs, we have learned an important fact and that is that if the American Indian approves of an herb, we can be sure that it has outstanding merit. The Indians knew all about influenza, and some of their people were stricken with it long before the great world war. But it was then not called influenza, but break-bone fever because the pain attending it produced the sensation of breaking bones, probably because of the unbearable tension and contraction of ligaments which, when temporarily relaxed in clonic (convulsive) spasms, produced the sensation that the bones were breaking.

We explain this because boneset immediately relieves that clonus and sets and rests the bones. Therefore it is a superb remedy for not only break-bone fever , but also for every other kind of fever man is subject to. In all cases of influenza, severe colds, chills and fever, the patient must be in bed warmly covered, and hot drinks of the infusion of boneset given in one half teacupful doses every half hour until a copious perspiration sets in. If it produces vomiting at first, so much the better. In that case wait until vomiting has completely subsided, then proceed until free perspiration is produced.

We have never known this herb to fail to overcome influenza and we are of the opinion that there would never be another death from this disease if boneset were at hand and freely used.

Another great flu remedy: For the treatment of fevers of all kinds, colds, and influenza, this remedy of elder flower and peppermint leaves is a safe, sure and speedy remedy. Aside from being anti-febrile, elder is an all around alterative, blood purifier and general systemic cleanser.

The great herbalist, Henry Box of Plymouth, England, says:

For colds, influenza, fevers, inflammation of the brain, pneumonia (inflammation of the lungs), stomach, bowels or any part, this is a certain cure. I have never known it to fail, even when given up, and at the point of death. It will not only save at the eleventh hour, but at the last minute of that hour. Besides, it is so safe and harmless that you cannot use it amiss.

This wonderful, wise old man had been a physician of herbs for over sixty years and was known as one of the great doctors of his time. The following tea can be very helpful.

Preparation:

The infusion for the tea is made as follows:

1/2 ounce elder flowers
1/2 ounce peppermint leaves (crushed)

1 1/2 pints boiling distilled water

Pour boiling water over the herbs, cover and allow to steep in a hot place twenty minutes. Strain and sweeten with honey, then drink the whole amount of tea as hot as possible while closely covered in bed. Cover a hot water bottle with a cloth or towel dipped in apple cider vinegar and place on the feet. In a few minutes there will be copious perspiration, and the pulse will slow down and the patient will sleep peacefully for hours. The elder flowers are alterative, diaphoretic, diuretic, aperient, sudorific, emetic, relaxant, calmative and soporific. The chemical constituents of elder flower are volatile oil, pectin, potassium chloride, potassium sulphate, sodium, magnesium, calcium salts and a small quantity of potassium nitrate. These substances, of course, all are organic and natural.

When taken alone, elder flowers are inclined to be emetic and somewhat nauseous to some people. This effect can be prevented by combining them with peppermint. Peppermint is stimulant, nervine, calmative, and antiemetic, which offsets the undesirable effects of the elder flower. This combination is world-famous as a great fever and cold remedy.

Another herbal combination that we use to counter to common cold is the Garlic Juice Plus Formula (Anti-Plague). This may be taken in large amounts if necessary, from a tablespoon full every hour to a tablespoon full every fifteen minutes. This herbal formula has aided countless people to become well in a very short period of time.

CONSTIPATION

See Appendix A, Bowel Cleansing and Nourishing as well as *Dr. Christopher s Guide to Colon Health.*

COUGH

Definition and Symptoms:

A cough is a sudden, violent expulsion of air from the lungs (the body trying to dislodge mucus from the breathing passages).

Causes:

Deranged stomach. The vitality of the system has become lowered by improper diet, loss of sleep, lack of exercise and fresh air, and improper elimination. The cough is caused by the inflamed throat or bronchial tubes. This inflammation causes mucus which the cough is trying to expel. If the stomach and system were kept in good condition, there would be very few colds. Improper clothing and bedding at night are often causes of colds the use of synthetic cloth instead of natural fibers such as cotton, wool, linen, and silk. The poisons and waste matter in the body make one more susceptible. When the system is kept in good health elimination is good, and the power of resistance is strong, coughs and colds are rare.

Herbal Aids and Preparation:

This old-time remedy for coughs is one of the best we have found. It is made by chopping up two large onions, placing into a pan and covering the onions with liquid honey, so the honey is at least one half inch above the onions in the pan. Low heat (under 130 degrees or below simmer) for several hours in a double boiler. Strain and press out the liquid and use it as a cough syrup. This can be from a teaspoon every fifteen minutes or half hour, as needed. Hold the syrup in the mouth and let it trickle down the throat slowly. For each pint of liquid honey used, add one ounce (more or less as desired) of licorice root powder or the same amount of horehound herb or wild cherry bark. Add the herb you choose to use when the honey and onions are put together at the beginning. Any one of these three mentioned herbs is a very fine expectorant and demulcent herb and is used to aid in breaking up phlegm and discharging it. This remedy is good for clearing out the lungs and bronchials and also disperses itself throughout the whole system with great benefit.

Coughs are highly misunderstood. Usually a sore throat and coughing are caused by the sinuses draining down the eustachian tubes, which is like pouring acid down the throat. In this case, to aid in clearing the sinuses, grate up horseradish root into small pieces and mix into apple cider vinegar until it is a thick paste. An easy way to do this is to blend the small chopped pieces of horseradish and apple cider vinegar in the blender until it is about the same texture as horseradish sauce from the store (but, of course, without the preservatives, etc.).

Inhaling this into the nose will help clear the sinuses to some extent, but the patient should take about a fourth or one eighth of the teaspoonful into the mouth, chew it and then swallow it. Do this three or more times a day, increasing the amount a little each three or four days. A half teaspoon or more can be taken at a time by an adult.

Additional Treatment:

It is very beneficial to massage the chest and across the back with Antispasmodic tincture and to take six drops or more of the antispasmodic tincture several times each hour with a little distilled water. In addition, give a fourth cup or more of tea made of equal parts of wood betony, spearmint, peppermint, and catnip. Give this two or three times a day.

For years we have used a fine combination of herbs to aid in longtime respiratory irritation of the lungs and bronchials. This is an aid in emphysema as well as other bronchial lung congestion such as bronchitis, asthma, tuberculosis, etc. For a child, a fourth cup or more two or three times a day is suggested. It is made up of marshmallow, mullein, comfrey, lobelia and chickweed in equal parts.

CROUP

Definition:

Croup is a childhood disease characterized by laborious and suffocative breathing and a harsh, brassy, crowing cough. Usually occurs at night, during the course of an upper respiratory infection.

Symptoms:

When the child takes a breath there is a whistling sound and often it sounds like he is strangling.

Cause:

Croup may be caused by the overeating of mucus-forming foods (including foods eaten by the mother who is nursing-such as dairy products), or by the overeating of any food, with fermentation in the stomach causing phlegm.

Herbal Aids:

Give the child a few drops of tincture of lobelia in catnip and peppermint tea, then a warm bath or hot foot bath, followed by a catnip tea enema.

Other Treatment:

Follow the bath with a thorough rubdown with olive oil, and apply Anti-Spasmodic tincture (or lobelia tincture) to the chest and back as a liniment. Keep the air moist a good vaporizer is a great help for quick relief. Keep the bowels open with mild laxative herbs and give a tea of catnip, cubeb berries, senna and black cohosh with a few drops of tincture of lobelia to relieve the spasms. Give by the teaspoon or tablespoon according to age every half hour until relief is obtained. The child should be kept on a fruit and fruit juice diet for a few days. An oatmeal and slippery elm gruel is also nourishing and helpful.

CUTS, ABRASIONS, BRUISES

Definition:

These are wounds to the skin. A cut severs the skin, such as is inflicted by a sharp object, an abrasion rubs and/or scratches the surface, such as the common scraped knee, and a bruise results from forceful pressure against some object, where the skin is not broken so the blood rushes to the damaged tissue beneath the surface.

Symptoms:

The appearance of these wounds are obvious. However,

certain cuts such as those that are deep and wide may require immediate attention by a doctor to prevent scarring. If the bleeding does not stop using the following methods, or if blood gushes in bright spurts, you should seek medical attention immediately.

Herbal Aids:

The old herbalists claimed that cayenne pepper should be poured directly into a fresh wound, to sterilize and stop the bleeding. Also, if a doctor is not available, apply fresh or dry comfrey root or leaf, powdered, to help stop the bleeding. The comfrey can be put right into the wound; if it is powdered, pour over the area, if fresh, tear up finely and apply. Fresh or dried comfrey can be applied directly over the damaged area just keep adding additional amounts as needed. Cover with gauze, bandage lightly to hold comfrey in place but so the area can breathe. Comfrey paste (see Burns) can also be applied directly over the damaged area as with burns. The Complete Tissue Formula may also be used to heal these conditions. Use the ointment externally and the capsules internally.

A wound, external or internal, will stop bleeding if the individual will drink a cup of water (preferably hot) with a teaspoon of cayenne pepper (red pepper) stirred into it. The bleeding will stop generally by the time a person can count to ten after drinking the cayenne tea. The cayenne equalizes the blood pressure from the top of the head to the feet. This keeps the pressure from the hemorrhage area so it will clot naturally, which it cannot do with heavy blood pressure pumping the blood rapidly at the hemorrhage area. Moistened chewing tobacco, shave grass, shepherds s purse, wild alum root, and yellow loosestrife will all aid in stopping bleeding and assist in healing, but comfrey is one of our favorites and should be in everybody s yard or in a flower pot in the apartment or house, or keep a good supply of the powdered leaf and root on hand. Bruises respond equally well to a pack of fresh, crushed comfrey, or the powdered leaves or roots made into a paste with water.

DIABETES

Definition, Symptoms, Causes:

The origin of this disease, as is known so far, can be traced back to derangement of the functions of the pancreas gland. Contributing factors, however, are undoubtedly severe nervous disturbances, or improper function of stomach, liver and bowels, and the use of dairy products. The patient feels tired and weak, usually complains about pains in the limbs, feeling depressed and down-hearted, and an abnormal thirst is often experienced. Dizziness and headaches are also common. The skin is dry and often itchy. The digestion is often upset, due to the abnormally increased appetite. The eyesight may be impaired or weak. The urine is generally very pale and plentiful. Sugar is generally present in the urine in greater quantities.

Herbal Aids:

For the continued thirst, flaxseed tea, with a small quantity of peppermint herb, may be used freely. The diet should be carefully watched. Dairy products, sugars and starches should be eliminated. Use unprocessed fruits, vegetables, grains, nuts and seeds. The bowels should be kept well regulated. Rest and sunshine are also beneficial.

We have an herbal formula named the Pancreas Formula (Panc-Tea) used to heal the pancreas and other affiliated glands which through malfunction cause high or low blood sugar; namely, diabetes or hypoglycemia. This combination has assisted many that have had hypoglycemia after six months or more of using two or three capsules, three times a day, six days a week. (All herbal aids give faster results in six days a week instead of seven, using the same day of the week of each week for the day of rest). Many have had a glucose tolerance test with a clean bill of health on the pancreas area after using this program. Many reports came in about heavy insulin users who continue using the insulin but, by watching litmus paper or other types of diabetic checking, have gradually tapered down on the insulin; and many, within a year of using two to three capsules three times a day, six days a week, have found complete relief. Of course, the closer a person stays on the mucusless diet and eliminates from the diet the unnatural sugars, daily products, soft drinks, candies, pastries, bread, etc., the quicker the results. The herbal formula is goldenseal, uva ursi, cayenne, cedar berries, licorice root and mullein. Another aid for Type 1 Diabetes is the Immucalm formula. This formula helps calm and strengthen the immune system. This is needed because this form of diabetes is also an auto-immune disorder and the immune system is attacking the beta cells in the pancreas.

DIARRHEA

Definition:

Diarrhea is the abnormal frequency and liquidity of fecal discharges.

Symptoms:

It is characterized by frequent morbid and profuse liquid discharges.

Causes:

Diarrhea has a number of causes: too much fruit, digestive upset, and stressful emotion are some. It may be the body ridding itself of toxins. It is the most severe form of constipation and should be dealt with immediately.

Herbal Aids:

Dr. H. C. Alfred Vogel (The Nature Doctor, Verlag, Switzerland: Bioforce) says: There is a little plant which will put an end to this unpleasant trouble almost without exception: Tormentil. Use this as a tea and use as needed.

An excellent and easy-to-find herb for diarrhea is the common wild and domestic sunflower leaf. Make up a tea of this and start giving a teaspoon a time. Increase the amount gradually if needed, but not too fast, as it will cause constipation if too much is taken.

The Lower Bowel Formula may be used to relieve constipation if present. If diarrhea persists or becomes worse, take a quarter cup of slippery elm gruel four times a day. This acts as a mild laxative but makes bowel movements more solid.

A real lifesaver is a rectal injection of oak bark tea, and also drinking the tea. This works in the most severe cases. We must always go back to the cause, after relieving the effect, by checking the diet.

Should the diarrhea be of a more serious nature, keep the child on nothing but teas for six, twelve, twenty-four hours or more, depending on the age of the child. The following herbs are suitable for this purpose: red raspberry, yarrow, oak bark, bayberry bark, garden sage, mullein, marshmallow, nettle, slippery elm, strawberry leaves, ginger, and plantain.

EARACHE

Definition:

Pain or aching in the ear.

Symptoms:

This can be a painful condition for all ages. Little babies rubbing and pulling on their ears are not able to tell you what is wrong, so be observant. Children and adults also suffer from the same condition, and can be handled in the same manner. Other symptoms include dizziness or loss of equilibrium.

Causes:

Sometimes earaches are caused by infection, cold in the head, a blow to the side of the head, a mucus buildup in the middle or inner ear, and many other causes.

Herbal Aids and Preparation:

The simple, old-fashioned aids are sometimes very fast in giving relief. We will give you a number of aids that have been used successfully for many years. Always treat both ears, even if only one aches.

Onion. Lightly bake a large onion, cut it in half while warm, bind one half of the onion over each ear. Hold bandage on with a nightcap, and leave on all night.

Garlic. Drop four to six drops of oil of garlic into each ear and plug with warm cotton. Also add four drops of the Nerve Formula (B&B) described in the formula index.

Chamomile. Use a fomentation over both ears of three parts of chamomile and one part of lobelia. Take two ounces orally every two waking hours. Leave the fomentation on the ears all night. Cover fomentation with plastic or oiled silk, etc.

Mullein. Use three to six drops of mullein oil in both ears several times each day. Insert it upon retiring for the night, and, as before, plug the ears with cotton. Place a fomentation over the ears all night of three parts mullein and one part lobelia. This oil may also be massaged under the ear to relieve pressure in the eustachian tube.

Lobelia. Place a few drops of warm tincture of lobelia into each ear and plug with cotton. Substitute with antispasmodic tincture or nervine tincture if needed.

Hops. Apply a flannel bag of hops and moist heat (a hot water bottle, never dry heating pad) over the affected area.

ECZEMA (AND OTHER FORMS OF DERMATITIS)

Definition:

Eczema is an inflammatory skin disease sometimes a rash with watery discharge or development of scales and crusts.

Symptoms:

The skin breaks out and itches with burning and stinging. Sometimes little pimples form which turn into water blisters. Usually the skin dries up into little scales and itches.

Causes:

The skin is a very important part of the body, it is an extra kidney, an extra set of lungs for breathing, and has many other functions. We should keep it in a good condition, important as it is, but we usually treat it shamefully. The skin should be bathed daily. This does not mean to use soap with each bathing, unless it is a natural type biodegradable liquid soap. Nearly all bar soaps do more damage to the skin than they aid it, by leaving residue of the soap to clog the pores. The pores are the doors and windows of the temple and must be kept open to let in oxygen (the breath of life) and to excrete toxins and waste.

A person who uses lots of mucus foods has a gluey, sticky type perspiration. When this individual sweats and the body is not cleaned regularly, the dried sweat clogs the pores. This is a beginning cause of dermatitis, or skin malfunction. In addition, as a nation we have fallen in love with easy to wash and iron synthetic clothes. These rob the body of the breath of life because man-made synthetic fibers do not breathe. Only natural fibers such as cotton, wool, linen, silk, etc., can allow the skin to breathe properly.

These are two of our big problems; the third one is a diet devoid of wholesome foods. We use man s prepared materials, called food, that have been contaminated and processed, and in so many cases, should be classified as junk food. All aids to fighting dermatitis work better and faster if we consider the first three things mentioned bathe regularly, return to natural fibers to wear, and eat wholesome foods.

Herbal Aids:

For eczema and other skin problems, use a fomentation over the irritated area made with chickweed tea and/or plantain, burdock root, Oregon grape root, and echinacea covered with plastic. Or bathe the area with the tea a number of times during the day. Chickweed or plantain ointment is an aid for small outbreaks. Drink a cup of the tea two or three times or more a day. To each cup of the tea you drink add three to six drops of tincture of lobelia.

A wonderful aid to relieve cases of dermatitis is found in the walnut family, using black walnut hulls, leaves or bark, English walnut, or butternut. Treat the skin malfunctions the same therapy as with number one.

Take one ounce of powdered goldenseal root and mix thoroughly with nine ounces of linseed (flax) oil. Use the medicinal linseed oil from the health food store or drug store, not linseed oil from the paint store or hardware store. Apply freely, externally. As an oral aid, use white poplar bark (also known as quaking aspen), one cup three times in a day.

For the most severe cases of skin diseases in the advanced stage, use a formula we have called The Complete Tissue Formula (BF&C), internally and externally. Make a tea of the following herbs: oak bark, marshmallow root, mullein herb, wormwood, lobelia, skull cap, comfrey root, walnut bark (or leaves), and gravel root. Soak the combined herbs in distilled water (at the rate of one ounce of the combined herbs to the pint of distilled water), for four to six hours. Simmer thirty minutes (do not boil), strain and then simmer the liquid down to one-half its volume. Example: one gallon of tea simmered down to two quarts of tea, which is called concentrated tea.

Preparation:

Soak flannel, cotton, or any white natural material. Wrap fomentation (soaked cloth) around the malfunctioning area and cover with plastic or wax paper, leave on all night six days a week and for as many weeks as needed until relief appears. Continue a week or two longer for severe cases. Drink one fourth cup of finished concentrated tea with three fourths cup of distilled water three times or more each day.

EYESIGHT, POOR

Definition:

Nearsightedness, astigmatism, farsightedness, cataracts, glaucoma, crossed-eyes, lazy eye, etc.

Symptoms:

Poor vision, blurred or distorted vision

Causes:

So many young children are wearing glasses today because, in many cases there is the weakness of the parents being handed down to the children. The excessive use of salt can cause loss of vision, as explained by Viktoras Kulvinskas in *Survival into 21st Century* (Omangod Press, Wettersfield, Conn.). The overuse of sugars leaches out the calcium from the veins in the eyes. Wearing glasses all the time keeps the sunshine filtered out of the eyes and this is a great loss, because the sunshine is a great doctor. Never, of course, look directly at the sun. Glasses should be used only when absolutely needed, and the rest of the time go without them.

Herbal Aids:

For a patient with cataracts or glaucoma, nearsightedness, farsightedness, eyes off-focus, use carrot juice, the mucusless diet, and the eyewash routine as follows. The Herbal Eyebright Formula is excellent for brightening and healing the eyes, and it has been known in some cases to remove the cataracts and heavy film from the eyes.

Make this into tea form and put into a glass eye cup. There will be a slight burning sensation from the cayenne in the eye at first, but there is nothing to be concerned about. Tip head back and apply the eye cup to eye. Exercise eye while doing this as though you were swimming under water. Do this three to six times a day. Drink ß cup of the tea a.m. and p.m.

The Bilbrite Eye Formula should be taken in conjunction with the eyewash formula for best results. Take three capsules three times daily.

Additional Treatments:

Use eye exercises to strengthen them. The less television that is watched, the better the eyes!

Carrot juice. A young man came to us seeking help because he wanted to become an Air Force Pilot with the government but was turned down because of bad eyesight. He had passed everything else with high grades, but the answer was still no, because of poor eyesight. When he asked the medical doctor if he could try again later, he was laughed at and told this condition could not be changed. He persisted and so was given a three-months return date. We had him clean his bowels, go on the mucusless diet after the three-day cleanse, and then drink one quart or more of freshly-made carrot juice each day, six days each week. He was to use nothing but distilled water on the seventh day. In three months he returned for another eye examination at the Air Force Agency, and this time was given the approval with a clean bill of health and good eyesight.

When there is poor eyesight, it is always good to use zonal foot therapy (reflexology), working on the corresponding eye area on the foot with good massage.

FEVERS

See Appendix C.

GLANDS, SWOLLEN

Definitions and Symptoms:

Some of the most important and mysterious parts of the body are the various glands. These select their required substances from which they synthesize new compounds. Upon the work of these secretions which the glands send forth into the body depend digestion, absorption and utilization of all food elements, and the very existence of cells. No physiological or mental activity is possible without them. In their absence, the body and its activities would cease to be. Manifestly, the glands cannot pick their required elements from the blood unless their progenitors were previously taken in the foods eaten.

The lymph vessels are fine tubes which accompany the blood vessels. They contain the lymph, a colorless, alkaline fluid, partly derived from the blood, partly from the juices of the partaken foods. To the lymph tubes belong the lymph nodes, which are distributed over the whole system, having been given the task of extracting poisonous substances from the lymph. The lymph travels through the whole body like the blood, gathers in larger and larger vessels, and finally flows into the large veins near the heart where it mixes with the blood, passes through the kidneys and lungs, and finally enters the heart as fresh new blood.

Causes:

The more toxic the poisons and mucus materials taken into the system, the more often the glands accumulate this bad waste from the lymph system and we have glandular swellings over various parts of the body. An impure blood stream, constipation and a generally toxic body condition cause the lymph nodes and glands to swell up and become painful. These may be on the neck, under the armpits, groin, etc.

Herbal Aids:

One of the finest combinations to keep the glandular system flowing free is three parts of mullein and one part lobelia. Use these two herbs as fomentation or as a poultice and put over the swollen gland. In most cases relief comes overnight. Continue using this nightly, until the condition is completely cleared. Also drink one-half cup of the mullein and lobelia tea three times each day until glands are back to normal. This combination is good for swollen tonsils, mumps, swollen breast from mastitis, swollen or injured testicles, etc.

Preparation:

To make a fomentation, first make the tea, using a teaspoon of dried herbs to a cup of distilled water or an ounce (two tablespoons approximately) to the pint of water. When the tea has steeped and has been strained, soak flannel or any cotton, wool, linen, silk of natural fiber in it. Place the sponged-out cloth over the swollen gland area. Cover with wax paper, oiled silk, plastic or other type of covering to keep the moisture going into the glandular area. Cover with dry toweling and leave on all night and continue using until healed.

We have seen many cases of mastitis and other swollen glands in various parts of the body given relief from the fomentation being used for one night alone. Some cases may take longer. Always remember the cause improper intake of foods.

Additional Treatments:

This procedure will give relief to the effect, but why not go to the cause, cleaning up the bowels and the blood stream, and following the mucusless diet for better health.

HEARING

Definition, Symptoms, Causes:

When a person cannot hear well, it may be from several causes, such as injury and concussion, nerve-loss, ears plugged with wax and/or debris.

Herbal Aids:

Dr. Christopher s Garlic Oil and the Nerve Formula (B&B). When this procedure is used as explained here, it can be an aid in assisting in improvement of poor equilibrium, failure of hearing, etc. With an eye dropper insert into each ear at night four to six drops of oil of garlic and four to six drops of the Nerve Formula and plug the ears cotton. Do this six days a week, four to six months, or as needed. On the seventh day, flush ears with a small ear syringe using warm apple cider vinegar and distilled water, half and half. This program has restored the hearing of many adults and children.

Preparation:

The Nerve Formula consists of blue vervain, black cohosh, blue cohosh, skullcap, and lobelia herb in equal parts using 90 proof or stronger alcohol as a base.

HICCUPS (OR HICCOUGHS)

Definition:

Hiccups are sudden inhalations of air caused by spasmodic contractions of the diaphragm.

Symptoms:

An irritation of the phrenic nerve causes the contractions of the diaphragm. Hiccoughs can at times become so serious they cause death, after a period of continued hiccoughing.

Causes:

This is generally caused by overloading food or drink into the stomach.

Herbal Aids and Preparation:

Relaxation is the most important thing for this condition, so drinking a mild nervine tea will help. Drinking a little orange juice is also helpful or take a teaspoon of onion juice. A few drops of antispasmodic tincture taken internally and rubbed on the chest area will often bring relief, as will a cayenne poultice on the chest area or black or blue cohosh tea.

A remedy that has proven very successful with us is to drink a few drops of Nerve Formula (B&B) given below. This is beneficial to have on hand at all times for hiccoughs, earaches, ringing in ears, etc. It is made as follows: Take one ounce each of blue cohosh, black cohosh, blue vervain, skullcap and lobelia, cut or powdered, and cover them in a quart-sized bottle, with one pint of grain alcohol 90 proof or stronger. Tighten the cap and shake this mixture three or more times each day for fourteen days. On the fourteenth day, strain, press out the liquid, filter through natural fiber cloth (cotton, wool, linen, etc.), never through synthetic cloth. Bottle this tincture in dark bottles or keep in a dark area, and you will find many uses for it when a good nervine or relaxant is needed.

INCURABLES

Definition:

Polio, infantile paralysis, curvature of the spine, muscular dystrophy, multiple sclerosis, leukemia and many others are labeled incurable conditions. The following program is one that uses only the natural wholistic routine of rebuilding malfunctioned areas with beneficial but harmless nontoxic procedures. These natural methods have been used since the time of Hippocrates, Galen, and other inspired teachers of health.

Symptoms and Causes:

We have many times made the statement There are no incur - able diseases, but at times there are incurable patients. The Creator has given herbs and wholistic therapies for every type of body malfunc- tion; and if they are used as described benefits will come, otherwise they can be of no aid.

No one can truly tell a patient he has just so many days, weeks, or months to live. The scriptures are plain in saying that everything moves in its time and season; there is an hour to be born and an hour to die. We have seen cases where the person was told that he had only a few days to live, many of these people are alive and well today, because they had faith to turn to the natural ways of healing and have been healed.

We have seen cases where the patients were lying helpless on the bed, so sickly they could not feed themselves, waiting for death at any moment. These people, by correctly utilizing the wholistic healing program, are alive, active and well today.

Even if a person appears near death and is suffering great pain, and perhaps his allotted time to go is near at hand, when the natural healing procedure is used the pain can be reduced and comfort given in their last hours. Every one of God s children is worthy of help to ease unbearable conditions with helpful but harmless natural aids.

This program has been used for many different malfunctions with great success in nearly every case: multiple sclerosis, muscular dystrophy, stroke, deteriorating bones, curvature of the spine, locked arthritic joints, tumors and cysts in nearly all parts of the body. We have seen great improvement, reduction in pain and often complete healing in cases supposedly incurable. As you read each step used in this program, analyze it and see if it can do anything but good. You will see that not one harmful thing is recommended.

Because of the length of Dr. Christopher s Incurables Program description, it is placed as Appendix D.

INFLUENZA, FLU

Definition:

An acute, infectious epidemic disease.

Symptoms and Causes:

Distressing fever, acute catarrhal inflammation of the nose, larynx, and bronchi, neuralgic and muscular pains, gastrointestinal disorder, and nervous disorders. These are followed by nervous prostration and great debility caused by excessive retention in the body of food wastes providing a feeding ground for these various bacteria and viruses.

Herbal Aids, Preparations, Additional Treatments:

See Appendix C, Fevers: Their Causes and Aids & The Cold Sheet Treatment.

INSECT STINGS AND BITES

Definition, Symptoms, Causes:

A sharp prick with an acute burning sensation. It is caused by the fine hairs in the stinging nettle; by the tail of the wasp, bee, etc.; from the head of gnats; from the claws of centipedes. Usually the sting causes a local, reversible inflammation. When the sting carries pollen, it may cause violent constitutional reactions in victims who are hypersensitive to that pollen, sometimes causing death.

Herbal Aids, Preparation:

Bruise with a mortar and pestle or juice in a juicer fresh plantain leaves and place over the sting or bite. Relief will generally come within a very short time, the pain and itch will stop and the swelling will leave. Rub the bruised leaves or juice over the exposed parts of the body, and it will discourage the insects from annoying you. The juice or crushed leaves of elderberry, walnut, lilac, and hounds tongue will assist in keeping bites and stings to a minimum.

Drink a nervine tea such as skullcap, black cohosh, wood betony or valerian and/or pennyroyal and parsley, taken with a few drops of tincture of lobelia, as often as needed.

It is recommended that one or more of the good herbs mentioned above be kept on hand at all times. Have the herbs in dry form which can be soaked in a little distilled water (plain tap water in a crisis) in tincture form or as an ointment.

When using the fresh herb, such as plantain that grows almost everywhere, take the freshly gathered herb leaves, root, blossoms, etc., and use a mortar and pestle to bruise and make the herb into a pasty form. If not equipped with mortar and pestle, use a spoon in a bowl, or a rolling pin on a board, a hammer on a solid surface. If you have a centrifugal juicer like an Acme, a Champion or a Norwalk with tritcherator and press, use these. Within a few minutes of using the plantain, the pain leaves and the swelling starts to recede.

We have gone on a house call where the hand and arm were swollen and up the arm was a red streak with a lump under the arm pit.

The individual had fainted with pain from the wasp sting and swelling. It was early spring and the plantain was not up, so I could not use it fresh. I put plantain ointment, about the size of a dollar, over the sting and within a half an hour the pain was gone. This was in the morning, and they reported back later that the swelling and red streak were gone by afternoon and this boy was out playing ball later that day.

A good scout is always prepared. You should have herbs on hand for these emergencies, as you never know when they are going to occur.

ITCH

Definition and Symptoms:

Local irritation of the skin that is often accompanied by inflamation and redness.

Causes:

Itch is caused by various germs or bacteria trying to clean the body through the pores of the skin rather than through the kidneys and the bowels, resulting in formation of pustules or rashes accompanied by intense itching.

Herbal Aids:

For itch and other skin problems, use a fomentation over the irritated area made with chickweed tea and/or plantain, burdock root, Oregon grape root, and echinacea covered with plastic. You can also, bathe the area with the tea a number of times during the day. Chickweed or plantain ointment is an aid for small outbreaks. Drink a cup of the tea two or three times or more a day. To each cup of the tea you drink, add three to six drops of tincture of lobelia.

A wonderful aid to relieve cases of dermatitis is found in the walnut family, using black walnut hulls or leaves or bark, English walnut, or butternut. Treat the skin malfunctions the same as with number one.

Take one ounce of powdered goldenseal root and mix thoroughly with nine ounces of linseed (flax) oil. Use only the medicinal linseed oil from the health food store or drug store, and apply freely, externally. Also use white poplar bark, also known as quaking aspen, one cup three times a day as an oral aid.

For the most severe cases of skin diseases in the advanced stage use our Complete Tissue Formula (BF&C) internally and externally. Make a tea of the following herbs: oak bark, marshmallow root, mullein, wormwood, lobelia, skullcap, comfrey root, walnut bark (or leaves) and gravel root.

Preparation:

Soak the combined herbs in distilled water, one ounce of the combined herbs to the pint of distilled water, for four to six hours, simmer thirty minutes (do not boil), strain and then simmer the liquid down to one-half its volume. Example: One gallon of tea simmered down to two quarts of tea, which is called concentrated tea.

Soak flannel, cotton, or any white material other than synthetic in the tea and wrap the fomentation (soaked cloth) around the malfunction area and cover with plastic or wax paper, leave on all night six days a week and for as many weeks as needed until relief appears. Then continue a week or two for severe cases. Drink one fourth cup of finished concentrated tea with three-fourths cup of distilled water three times or more each day.

JAUNDICE

Definition:

Jaundice is due to absorption of bile into the blood vessels, a disposition of bile pigment in the skin and mucous membrane.

Symptoms:

The patient appears yellow. Symptoms are yellow skin and whites of eyes, bitter taste in mouth, constipation, urine is dark, slight fever, headache, and dizziness.

Causes:

Jaundice, hepatitis, and contagious hepatitis stem from a liver/ gall bladder malfunction. This is the cause, but the root cause is poor diet.

Jethro Kloss (*Back to Eden*, Back to Eden Publishing) gives the following on jaundice:

> Causes: Obstruction of the bile. When the bile gets into the blood or circulation it causes the skin all over the body to become yellow, as well as the whites of the eyes. The bile does several important things: It neutralizes the gastric juice which would otherwise interfere with intestinal digestion; it alkalinizes the food and enables the system to take care of it; it has a special effect on the fatty foods. Deficient bile is the cause of constipation. Derangement of the stomach, liver and bowels is the cause of this ailment, and of course, these troubles arise from errors in diet.

Herbal Aids:

One of the safest and fastest methods of reversing these conditions is to follow the three-day cleanse routine as follows: drink apple juice each waking hour, swishing (chewing) each mouthful of the juice in the mouth, so the saliva mixes with it thoroughly. A child eight years old or older can generally use an eight-ounce glass each hour, younger children in proportion. No other food is used. If desired, on the half-hour distilled water can be used. During each day of the three days, take one tablespoon or more of sweet-tasting, extra virgin cold pressed olive oil. To take away the oily taste, eat an apple or chew juice well right after the oil. (See Appendix B.)

Give the patient the Lower Bowel Formula several times a day to keep the bowels clear. This is a very important part of the program keeping the bowels free. One way to help is to start the day off with eight ounces or more of prune juice. Any brand from the grocer s shelf is good, as long as no preservatives have been added.

During each day have the patient take one half cup (more or less according to age) of a Liver and Gallbladder Formula (Barberry LG) three times a day. One of the most effective formulas we have recommended for many years is: three parts barberry root or substitute Oregon grape root or rocky mountain grape root, and one part of wild yam. If wild yam is not available, substitute two parts of sweet fennel seed.

During acute stages of jaundice (hepatitis), use a castor oil fomentation over the liver and gall bladder area (right side, lower rib cage and across abdomen). Massage castor oil in a circular clockwise motion over the area, using it liberally, or soak a flannel cloth in castor oil, squeeze out excess and cover area. After the castor oil is applied either by massage or fomentation (the latter is better), cover the area, flannel and all, with a hot wet towel. Keep a hot water bottle or a moist-type heating pad over the area for a half hour to an hour several times daily. Repeat the entire program from time to time until condition is cleared. Then stay on the mucusless diet, use plenty of carrot and other type juices and drink one ounce of steam distilled water per each pound of body weight each day.

LEUKEMIA

Definition and Symptoms:

According to Dorland s *The American Medical Dictionary* (Philadelphia and London: W. B. Saunders Co.):

> Leukemia: A fatal disease of the blood-forming organs, characterized by a marked increase in the number of leukocytes and their precursors in the blood, together with enlargement and proliferation of the lymphoid tissue of the spleen, lymphatic glands, and bone marrow. The disease is attended with progressive anemia, internal hemorrhage (as in the retina, etc.) and increasing exhaustion. Leukemia is classified clinically on the basis of (1) the duration and character of the disease acute or

chronic; (2) the type of cell involved myeloid (myelogenous), lymphoid (lymphogenous) or monocyclic; (3) increase or non-increase in the number of abnormal cells in the blood-leukemic or aleukemic (subleukemic) etc, over three pages of details of the effects.

Causes:

We have a different approach of healing; namely, going into the cause of the problem. Using non-toxic, non-poisonous, non-habit-forming aids to clean up the basic cause of malfunction, we clean the bowel, and strengthen, rebuild and purify the blood stream. With herbal aids and food we rebuild the nerves, the muscles, bones and tissue by properly feeding these areas with rich herbal nutrients.

The cause of leukemia is based on inherent weaknesses (sins of the parents to the third and fourth generations). These weaknesses are sins of commission or omission but these weak conditions can be strengthened and the body rebuilt by using the Incurables routine (see Appendix D).

LICE (BODY)

Definition:

Louse is a general name for various degraded parasitic insects; the true lice that infest mammals belong to the suborder *Anoplura Capitus*, or head louse; *P. Corporis*, the body or clothes louse; and *Phthirius*, or crab louse which lives in the hair upon the pubis, and the eye lashes and eye brows.

Symptoms:

The causal organisms of typhus fever, relapsing fever, trench fever, and possibly plague are transmitted by the bites of lice or mites.

Head lice will never stay around the body that is completely healthy, with no toxins or accumulations of mucus. Lice and all body vermin are scavengers and cannot exist long with clean healthy cells.

Keep the bowels clean, stay on a mucusless diet, bathe daily, and lice will not appear.

Herbal Aids:

When lice are present, use an infusion of six parts hyssop, one part walnut leaves or inner bark, one half part cinnamon bark powder, one half part cloves powder, one half part lobelia, and one half part ginger.

Dosage: a half cup (more or less according to age) three times in a day, taken orally. Make a fomentation over the head with the same formula, and in other areas infected; covering the fomentation with a plastic or rubber cap at night. Do this six days a week as many weeks as needed to clear up the condition.

For quick relief (working on the effect), bathe the head or body parts covered with lice with straight apple cider vinegar, oil of garlic or walnut (leaf, bark or nut husk) tea.

Additional Treatment:

When lice are detected in the family, see that in addition to working on the cause (cleaning the bowel and blood stream) and staying on a mucusless diet, work on the effect itself as suggested here. See that fresh clothes inner and outer clothing are changed daily . All of these clothes should be washed with a good biodegradable soap with a cup or more of apple cider vinegar added to each washerful of clothes. Change the bed linen each day. Spray the room with tea made of six parts chaparral, three parts black walnut leaf or bark, one part lobelia and to each pint of the spray add some lavender oil or oil of mint to give fragrance.

We must remember one thing, a clean house and clean body are not to the liking of our scavenger friends, lice, mites, fleas, etc.

MEASLES (RED AND GERMAN)

Definition:

Measles are a contagious eruptive fever with cold and catarrhal symptoms, due to a filterable virus (germs and bacteria surging out of the body through the skin) measles is one of nature s methods of housecleaning.

Symptoms of Red Measles:

The period of incubation is about two weeks, and the disease begins with fever, chills, often inflammation or reddening of eyelids or the membranes lining the eyelid, severe head cold frequently bronchitis causing cough and frontal headache. The eruption appears on the fourth day on the forehead, cheeks and back of the neck, then spreads over the body. It consists of small dark pink or rosy-red blotches in crescent shapes, often blending together, and the appearance of red spots surrounded by white areas in the mucous membrane of the mouth. In three or four days the eruption gradually fades, followed by a flaking or scaling of the area. The symptoms increase with the eruptions and decrease with their disappearance. Convalescence begins in the second week. The disease is extremely contagious and affects chiefly the young, and one attack usually confers immunity. Measles can lead to complications such as pneumonia and other lung problems, ear and eye infections.

Symptoms of German Measles:

German measles are not quite so severe as red measles, although they can be dangerous to a pregnant woman and the unborn child. After an incubation period of one to three weeks, the disease German measles begins with a slight fever and catarrhal symptoms, sore throat, pain in the limbs, and the appearance of an eruption of red papules similar to those of measles but lighter in color, not arranged in crescentic masses, and disappearing without scaling or flaking within a week.

Causes:

According to Dr. Kloss, measles are merely the system s attempt to cleanse itself of impurities.

Herbal Aids:

If the child is slow in breaking out, give a good hot bath. It is important to clean out the bowels, so give the patient a warm catnip tea enema each day. Put him to bed and give a tea made of equal parts of yarrow, pleurisy root and valerian root or catnip. Give this tea freely to produce perspiration which will also lower the fever. Red sage, red raspberry leaf or camomile teas are also excellent for a patient with measles. Another pleasant herbal tea made of equal parts catnip, raspberry leaf, and peppermint leaf, can be given freely throughout the day. It is best to keep the room dark so that the eyes will not become irritated. In the event the patient s eyes do become sore, bathe them two or three times a day with a tea made of equal parts of eyebright, raspberry leaf, and goldenseal. If the patient complains of itching, bathe or sponge the skin with a tea made of yellow dock and burdock root and/or goldenseal. Adding a little apple cider vinegar to a tub of bath water is also helpful.

Additional Treatment:

Guard the patient against bronchial troubles and earache and have him drink plenty of liquids distilled water , herbal teas, as recommended, and fruit juices. The diet should be simple, with plenty of fresh ripe fruit, fruit juices and fresh vegetable juice. One very good juice combination is carrot juice with celery, spinach and parsley juice added to taste. See also Appendix C, The Cold Sheet Treatment.

MUMPS

Definition:

A contagious childhood disease with inflammation of the glands around the tonsils and salivary glands.

Symptoms:

After an incubation period of about three weeks, the symptoms appear with fever, headache, and pain beneath the ear. Soon there develops a tense, painful swelling in the parotid region, which interferes with chewing and swallowing (both actions become very painful). After a few days to a week the symptoms gradually disappear. Sometimes the submaxillary and other salivary glands are involved, and occasionally the testicles become swollen.

Causes:

Mumps are the result of toxic mucus accumulations in the body.

Herbal Aids:

As quickly as evidences of mumps appear, use a fomentation of three parts mullein herb and one part lobelia (the Glandular System Formula) around the neck and swollen area. Cover this with plastic and a cloth or towel over the plastic to be more comfortable and also to hold in the heat. Replace fomentation each half hour or each hour for the day and leave it on all night.

In addition to using the fomentation on the neck area, also have the child drink a half cup (more or less according to age) of the mullein and lobelia tea, three or more times a day.

Other Treatment:

With mumps, as with all fever diseases, use the fever routine as explained in Appendix C at the back of this book.

NERVOUS, HIGH-STRUNG, HYPERACTIVE CHILDREN

Causes:

One of the doctors speaking at a recent national health convention just ahead of me stated in plain terms: For hyperactive children that are almost impossible to handle, do just one thing. This one procedure has been in clinics and has been proven to work. Take all junk food away from the child, feed him wholesome and proper food and there will be improvement within weeks.

This has been our teaching for years. Some years ago, a woman brought into our Salt Lake City office two brothers who appeared to be trying to kill each other. An older person had to be with them twenty-four hours a day to keep them from seriously injuring one another. As the boys were brought in, the poor mother had a firm hand on one arm of each boy, and was holding them apart as they were screaming at each other. She told us that the family doctor, a child specialist, and psychiatrists could do nothing with them. We put the boys on our mucusless diet, gave them some relaxant tea (The Nerve Combination), and in a couple of months they came in arm in arm, talking like school chums. The mother was so thrilled she had to bring them in for us to see the miraculous change. Please, let s get back to eating right and helping this next generation find peace.

Herbal Aids:

For small children, give a tea made of peppermint, spearmint and catnip, two or three times a day.

Additional Treatment:

Use the Relax-Eze Formula comprised of black cohosh, capsicum, hops flowers, lady s slipper, lobelia, skullcap, valerian wood betony and mistletoe. The suggested adult dose would be one to three cups of the tea, or two to three capsules three times a day, taken with a cup of celery juice or steam distilled water.

NOSEBLEEDS

Definition and Symptoms:

A nosebleed is a hemorrhage from the nose syn., epistaxis (from one side), epistaxis bilateral (both sides).

Causes:

Unless it is from injury, nosebleed results from a calcium deficiency. It is caused by the rupture of a small vessel in the nose due to pressure in the head. There are many causes for nosebleeds, but the weakness stems from calcium deficiency. Of course, it does not matter how much calcium is in the body if one is hit in the nose with a good blow; bleeding will start.

Herbal Aids:

A teaspoon of cayenne in a cup of water, hot preferred, taken internally will stop most nosebleeds quickly. In an emergency such as this we use cayenne. A teaspoon of cayenne pepper in a glass of water and drunk right down will stop a nosebleed in nearly every instance, by the time you can count to ten. This is not a miracle; it is the principle of the cell stimulant cayenne traveling through the entire blood stream and regulating the pressure so the pressure of the flow is the same in the feet as in the head or any other part of the body. This takes the heavy pressure off the hemorrhaging area and allowing a quick coagulation.

One of our very finest herbal foods is our Herbal Calcium Formula (Calc-Tea) which consists of comfrey root, horsetail grass, oat straw, and lobelia. Make this into a tea, using one teaspoon of combined herbs to cup of distilled water morning and one evening or two or three capsules two or three times per day.

If the nose bleeds often, the veins, capillaries and tissue often will be strengthened by inhaling a small amount of bayberry bark or oak bark tea up into the nose. If desired, use an atomizer to spray it up. Another method is to take the bayberry bark or oak bark powdered and with a small straw blow a very small amount of the powder up the nose each day, until healed. Do not blow too much of the powder up the nose or it will plug up the area. Drink a small amount, one-fourth cup more or less, of the bayberry or oak bark tea each day until the condition is under control.

RINGWORM

Definition and Symptoms:

Ringworm is caused by a fungus and is characterized by ring-shaped itching patches. Patches of round, itching rash cover the affected area. The very word of ringworm causes some people to shudder with fear, because they know how quickly it can spread over an area.

Causes:

Ringworm will never break out unless there is a toxic condition in the system. Look always to the inside problem while working on the effect, that is the external irritation.

Herbal Aids:

Make a strong tea of three parts plantain, three parts of yellow dock, and one part lobelia (or add tincture of lobelia to the tea) and foment the afflicted area each night, covered with plastic, six nights a week and continue on until healed.

Make a strong tea of sarsaparilla, three parts; black walnut leaves or bark, three parts; and one part lobelia. Use the same directions as in Number 1 on ringworm.

Make a garlic paste of fresh, chopped, grated or finely cut garlic one part, and petroleum jelly one part. Apply a generous amount over the afflicted parts, cover with gauze and leave on all night. During the day, massage with oil of garlic three or four times.

Use a strong decoction of oak bark; it can be white or tanner s, black, scarlet, red or western scrub oak. Make a fomentation and use as suggested in Number 1.

This will be used with the same directions as Number 1, but use a strong tea (decoction) of black walnut or English walnut or butternut bark and use as directed.

Massage the infected area three to six times a day with tincture of lobelia and olive oil half and half, and apply the tincture or oil on gauze and leave on all night.

Additional Treatment:

The six different aids listed above are for the effect or external relief. Be sure and clean up the cause, the toxic conditions in the body, and keep it clean with herbal laxatives and the mucusless diet, so there will be no recurrence. (See Appendices A and B.)

STIFF NECK

Definition and Symptoms:

Inability to move neck without pain and/or stiffness.

Causes:

Vertebrae in upper cervical thrown out, cold in neck, etc.

Herbal Aids:

The Complete Tissue Formula (BF&C) is the most complete formula for this condition of a stiff neck. As the fomentation penetrates into the area, it will relax the muscles and feed the nerves so the bone structure (vertebra) will adjust itself. At the same time it will build up the blood circulation to carry off waste materials, as well as feed the painful area with herbal food to put it into a healthy state of self healing.

When this formula is not available, use hot and cold fomentations, five or ten minutes of each; this will work on the effect but the Complete Tissue Formula will go to the cause.

To prepare the Complete Tissue Formula, make a tea of the following herbs oak bark, marshmallow root, mullein herbs, wormwood, lobelia, skullcap, comfrey root, walnut bark (or leaves), and gravel root. Soak the combined teas in distilled water (at the rate of one ounce of combined herbs to a pint of distilled water), then, soaking four to six hours, simmer thirty minutes, strain and then simmer the liquid down to 1/2 its volume and add 1/4 vegetable glycerine (if desired). Example: One gallon of tea simmered (not boiled) down to two quarts and add one pint of glycerine.

Soak flannel, cotton, or any white material other than synthetics. Wrap the fomentation (soaked cloth) around the malfunctioning area and cover with plastic to keep it from drying out. Leave on all night six nights a week, week after week, until relief appears.

Severe cases: Drink 1/4 cup of finished concentrated tea with 3/4 cup of distilled water three times in a day.

STY

Definition and Symptoms:

Inflammation of one or more of the sebaceous glands of the eyelids. Painful and swollen eyelids.

Causes:

Toxic poison accumulation.

Herbal Aids:

To give aid to healing a sty on the eyelid, make a fomentation of sarsaparilla root and apply over the eye.

Place a fomentation of mullein leaves, red raspberry leaves, goldenseal, slippery elm, lobelia and marshmallow root over the eye. Apply a fresh application for one hour at a time, three or more times a day, or leave on all night, until healed.

The Herbal Eyewash Formula. This formula is excellent for brightening and healing the eyes, and it is known to remove the cataracts and heavy film from the eyes. It includes bayberry bark, eyebright herb, goldenseal root, red raspberry leaves, and cayenne. Make this into tea form and put into a glass eye cup. There will be a slight burning sensation when using the cayenne in the eye at first, but there is nothing to be concerned about. Tip head back and apply the eye cup to eye. Exercise eye while doing this as though you were swimming under water. Do this three to six times a day. Drink 1/2 cup morning and evening. This formula has aided many sty cases.

TONSILLITIS

Definition:

Tonsillitis is the inflammation of the tonsils, acute catarrhal infection, redness and swelling, often the result of overworking them. Tonsils, many authorities say, are the first line of defense. Their job is to control the entrance of large armies of germs into the body.

Tonsils are the filtering system for the reproductive organs and are needed by the body, or the Creator would not have installed them in the first place. As a person goes from childhood into adulthood through the stage of puberty, the young people making this transition will be easier to live with if they still have their tonsils. The girls will have easier menstrual periods and the boys less chance for prostrate malfunction and will have a better teenage life.

We have ten fingers, but if we got infection in one of them, we would not cut it off until we tried to clear up the infection. As soon as the tonsils become swollen with infection the first thing we think of is to have the tonsils cut or burnt out, without trying to save them. Use our suggested program and keep the individual in a whole state, as the Creator intended!

Symptoms:

Dr. Kloss describes the symptoms as follows: Chilly feeling, fever, throat swollen, practically closed with soft palate hanging at the tongue. The throat and mouth are dry, and then soon lots of poisonous mucus accumulates. The tonsils are swollen and red in color. Small ulcers appear on the tonsils. Often the glands of the neck swell.

Herbal Aids:

With tonsillitis we use the Glandular Formula three parts mullein and one part lobelia. In addition to drinking the mullein and lobelia tea and applying the fomentation, use an abundance of red raspberry tea, as much as can be taken for three days. Use no foods on these days except unsweetened vegetable and fruit juices.

When the tonsils swell up and are sore and painful, the first thing we think of is to remove them. We saw a picture recently of seven or eight children spread out on a king-sized bed, all with wrapped-up throats. The caption explained that the family got a bargain by having them all operated on at once for tonsillectomies.

Here was a group of children who had lost a very valuable organ the Lord put into the body. It was not put there by mistake or carelessness, but because it was needed. This organ is the filtering system for the body, and when removed leaves us with a weaker system.

A girl with her tonsils intact will have an easier time through puberty and her menstrual cycles than she will if they have been removed. Delivery of babies is much easier for women who still have their tonsils, because of less toxic waste in the body.

The young boy with his tonsils intact will have better seed for reproducing and less chance of prostate problems because of a cleaner blood stream. To repeat, we have ten fingers and if we get infection in one of them we would not think of chopping it off without trying to heal the finger first. We only have two tonsils and, when there is a little infection in them, how foolish to cut or burn them out! As stated earlier, let s save these tonsils for better, stronger and more peaceful generations to come.

Additional Treatment:

When the tonsils become enlarged or inflamed, clean up the bowels, go off solid foods, go on the three-day cleansing program (see Appendix B).

TOOTHACHE

Definition:

Decay of teeth: decomposition due to lack of live organic atoms in the food to nourish the teeth.

Symptoms:

Pain or a dying in one or more teeth, sometimes accompanied by swelling of the gums.

Cause:

Tooth problems start several generations back. The weakness of calcium deficiency is passed from parent to child. By following the same parental pattern of poor food selection, each new crop of babies becomes weaker. While the baby is being carried in the womb, Mother Nature is interested in that which is being produced more than the one producing. She is continually trying to upgrade humans and animals by drawing on the mother to supply the child. How often do we hear the expression, W ell, I m carrying another child, that means more varicose veins and loss of more teeth. I don t see why mothers have to suffer this way. Please don t blame the Lord for these conditions, rather blame the use of pastries, soda pop, candy, sugar, ice cream, etc. The sugar in these products leaches the calcium out of the body. Pregnancy is a strain on body calcium, because the mother must have enough calcium in her body for both her and the baby being formed, and later for nursing. If there is not enough calcium for her, because of this leaching process by the sugar (of past and present), the fetus draws on the mother s body. The calcium it now takes is from the bones, muscles, and the teeth, etc. Sometimes so much is taken from the mother that she will, after a number of babies, have bone and muscle problems from a great lack of calcium.

When a child is being formed and there is not enough calcium supplied to the fetus, the jaw of the child will not form fully. It will be narrow instead of broad. When it is time for the child to cut teeth, they cannot come in straight because of a crowded jaw space. So naturally, they will come in crooked. Later, as there is not enough room for the wisdom teeth, they must often be extracted before coming through. When the day comes that the jaw is adequately large and well-shaped to accommodate all thirty-two teeth without crowding them to crookedness, and the wisdom teeth can remain until old age (and in comfort), it will mean we humans have gained enough wisdom to keep them!

The basic cause of calcium loss, of course, as mentioned, is leaching out the calcium with sugars and a toxic body condition. Nearly all tooth decay comes from the blood stream, saliva, and the inside of the teeth, not only from the external surface. The teeth deteriorate but it is from the enamel-destroying toxic saliva which is a result of an impure or toxic blood stream. If a child has good wholesome food and has been given a good solid start in life with a full healthy set of teeth and jaws, he can go through life without tooth problems. The condition of perfect teeth is, of course, dependent upon a continual use of wholesome and proper foods.

Herbal Aids:

Calcium is a must throughout life. It is needed for the formation of good teeth and strong bones. Children need calcium if bones and teeth are to grow strong and well-formed. Adults need an adequate amount of calcium every day. During periods of pregnancy and lactation, women require much more calcium than normal, as they must also furnish extra calcium for the baby.

Botanical or herbal sources for calcium are arrow root, comfrey, camomile, chives, dandelion root, flaxseed, horsetail grass, nettle, okra pods, oat straw, plantain, shepherds purse (and, of course, eat good foods rich in calcium). The Herbal Calcium Formula (Calc-Tea) and Kid-e-Calc are also designed to provide adequate calcium and the trace minerals needed to absorb it.

Additional Treatment

Another type of natural calcium is found in the use of eggshells. A chicken consumes grit and sandy materials, and these materials go into and through the gizzard into the blood stream. Then these calcium-type materials are taken from the blood stream to form the egg shell. After breaking the eggshell open, be careful to pull out the small membrane that lines the shell. This membrane is high in cholesterol and it is wise to eliminate it. Dry the shells at room temperature or under 130 degrees F. When thoroughly dry, powder the shells in a blender, nut mill or with a rolling pin. When the powder from one dozen eggshells is ready and finely powdered, cover with one pint of apple cider vinegar or one pint of lemon juice (lemon juice will sour and spoil quicker than the apple cider vinegar). Mix the eggshell powder and liquid in a large container, because the chemical reaction will cause the solution to foam.

For the adult, use two or more tablespoons (or add to distilled water, tea or juice if desired) and for children in proportion. Some people like to add a tablespoon of honey for each tablespoon of the vinegar-calcium mix, as this is a great help in adjusting the hydrochloric acid balance in the body as well as feeding calcium to the system.

WARTS AND/OR MOLES

Definition:

An elevation of the skin, more rarely of the mucous membrane, formed by hypertrophy of the papillae.

Symptoms:

Generally raised, darkened areas on the body.

Causes:

Warts and moles are usually the result of a nutritional deficiency and they should be treated internally, as well as externally.

Herbal Aids:

The warts, moles and skin blemishes are helped externally and are often cleared up by using the white milk from dandelions and/or from milkweed. Applying castor oil or garlic oil to the area several times a day and taping a piece of gauze soaked with this oil over the wart during the night will aid in clearing the condition. The use of a clove of garlic cut in half (or mashed or grated) and kept over the wart all night until it is gone has aided many. Black walnut tincture and the Nerve Formula have been used with such success that a number of people swear by them. The combination tinctures consists of blue vervain, black cohosh, blue cohosh, skullcap and lobelia herbs in equal parts, using ninety proof or stronger alcohol as a base.

Additional Treatment:

Use the mucusless diet and add plenty of raw carrots, kelp, dulse, or seaweed and onions to the diet.

WHOOPING COUGH

Definition:

Whooping cough is an infectious catarrhal inflammation of the air passages.

Symptoms:

Symptoms are violent, convulsive coughs consisting of several expirations followed by a loud, sonorous whooping inspiration. This is generally a children s disease and begins with spasmodic coughing spells. The face reddens and the eyes bulge. Sore throat and often vomiting may occur. After an incubation period of about two weeks, the catarrhal stage begins with a slight fever, sneezing, running at the nose, and a dry cough. In a week or two the paroxysmal stage begins with the peculiar whoop or crowing cough which frequently induces vomiting. This stage lasts from three to four weeks and is followed by a stage of decline during which the paroxysms grow less frequent and less violent, and finally cease. Advanced stages develop into bronchopneumonia.

Causes:

Whooping cough is a rapid accumulation of mucus in the throat, which causes choking and may cause death if not cleared. Eliminate the mucus as fast as possible.

Herbal Aids and Additional Treatment:

Lobelia herb or tincture used as a fomentation, as well as a few drops internally every few minutes, works well. To cut the phlegm, use a bayberry or oak bark tea as a gargle and swallow after gargling. Use a mixture of garlic with cayenne and honey every few minutes to help clear the throat. Make an infusion of thyme and use a tablespoon of thyme infusion and a tablespoon of honey, mixed together, and give when the cough is troublesome.

Another good herbal remedy for whooping cough is:

1/2 ounce hyssop
1/2 ounce red raspberry leaves
1/2 ounce turkey rhubarb
1/4 ounce bayberry bark
1/2 ounce thyme

Simmer the first four herbs slowly in 1 1/2 pints of distilled water for fifteen minutes, pour over the thyme and steep 1/2 hour (covered), strain.

Dosage: One teaspoon or more, as needed. Be sure to keep the feet warm and dry. Massage oil of garlic into the soles of the feet. Oil of garlic is good to have on hand at all times.

If you have fresh pennyroyal, squeeze out the juice, sweeten half and half with honey and take a teaspoon to a tablespoon of this mixture with each coughing spasm, or make a strong tea with the dry herb and use the same dosage as above.

The old time herbalist, Dr. Shook, had very effective aids for this condition as follows: He said to mix fresh garlic juice with olive oil or anhydrous lanolin, and rub on the throat, chest and between the shoulder blades. This gives great relief. He gives a formula as a specific for whooping cough: two ounces marshmallow root, two ounces garden thyme, one quart distilled water. Slowly simmer the herbs in the distilled water until reduced to one pint, strain, press, return liquor to saucepan and add two pounds brown sugar (substitute honey if desired), simmer five minutes. Skim off scum as it rises, cool, bottle and keep in cold place. Dose: For young children, one teaspoonful as needed for cough. Older children: two or three teaspoonfuls, according to age. Adults: one tablespoon every two or three hours. This is a merciful remedy in paroxysmal whooping cough; it gives almost instant relief. If this remedy is used persistently, it will eliminate the cough quickly and effectively.

In our own text, School of Natural Healing (Christopher Publications, Inc., P.O. Box 412, Springville, Utah), are a number of remedies. To cite a few of them: Lobelia herb or tincture used in fomentation, together with a few drops internally every few minutes works well. To cut the phlegm use a bayberry or oak bark tea as a gargle (swallow after gargling). Use crushed garlic with cayenne and honey every few minutes to help clear the throat. Red clover tea used often is beneficial. A half teaspoon or more of oil of garlic used often is a fine aid in relief of whopping cough. Mix one teaspoon of thyme, two teaspoons mistletoe, one teaspoon of lobelia in a pint of water. Infuse and strain. The dosage is one tablespoon each hour, or as needed. For children, adjust according to age.

We are including a number of herbal combinations to give you a large variety of herbs to choose from when some are not available.

The following is a good formula for this condition:

1 ounce slippery elm
1 ounce boneset
1 ounce licorice
1 ounce flaxseed or linseed
1 pint blackstrap molasses

Preparation: Simmer the herbs for twenty minutes in one quart of water, strain and stir in the molasses while hot. Sweeten with honey. Dosage: One tablespoon as required.

When nothing else is available, have the child drink as many cups of warm water as possible. Put the finger down the throat and have the child throw up. This will at times break loose the phlegm and bring it up. In addition, use lobelia tea and/or some tincture of lobelia in the warm water. This will help in cutting the phlegm and also in regurgitating.

WORMS

Definition:

Pinworms, tapeworms, and roundworms are parasites existing in the intestinal tract. The three most common types of worms found in the body are: the thread or seat worms (*Oxyurix vermicularis*), the roundworm (*Ascares lumbricoides lumbrici* , and the tapeworm (*Taeince-taenia solium, Bothriocephalus latus*). There are other less-common worms that enter the body, such as hookworms *(Ancylostoma duodenal*, *Nectar Americanus*) and those of unclean pork (*Tricchinella spiralis*), which thrive upon various conditions of filth and degeneration.

Symptoms:

Restlessness at night, picking the nose, gritting the teeth, itching at anus, dry cough, etc. Worms sometimes cause spasms, fits or convulsions.

Causes:

Poor diet, poor hygiene, and constipation are usually the problem. Worms are found when the stomach is deranged from eating improper foods. Worms are the effect. The cause of the worms is improper diet the lack of wholesome foods and heavy mucus and starchy food intake. To work on the effect and rid the body of worms is like killing the flies and leaving the garbage which has attracted them in the same foul condition.

Herbal Aids:

A simple remedy for a mild case of worms is to use pumpkin seeds. It is best when fresh seeds are used. To make the infusion, steep one ounce of crushed seeds for fifteen to twenty minutes in a pint of boiling hot water. Dosage: One teacupful or more (up to one pint daily), six days a week for one to three weeks. Also eat one to two ounces of the pumpkin seeds each day.

Another seed aid is to combine the following:

1 part pumpkin seeds, crushed
1 part watermelon seeds, crushed
1 part cucumber seeds, crushed

Dosage: Take one pint of emulsion (two ounces of seeds triturated in honey and distilled water) in doses at two hour intervals; or take one to two tablespoons of the crushed seeds in honey, syrup, etc., in three doses at two hour intervals.

The patient should fast during this treatment, then take an appropriate cathartic several hours after the last dosage such as senna tea or preferably the lower bowel formula. Use this procedure at least three days in a row.

One of our favorite worm formulas is as follows:
1 part pink root powder
1 part burdock root powder
1 part black walnut leaves powder
1 part male fern powder
1 part pomegranate root bark powder
1 part wormwood powder
1 part lobelia

Dose: Mix the above herbal powders together and give the patient 1/2 teaspoon of the powder in sorghum molasses or honey. Take each morning and night for three days. On the fourth day, drink one cup of three parts senna tea and one part peppermint tea, wait two days and repeat, two times.

Additional Treatment

To clean up the unsavory toxic condition that has attracted the worms, follow the instructions in Appendix A. See that the patient has three or more bowel movements each day.

Start feeding the patient the mucusless diet with plenty of whole, uncracked, presoaked, low-heated grains. Also, fruits, vegetables, nuts and seeds. By using this procedure we are getting to the cause, cleaning it up so there will be no recurrence. Be sure the patient drinks at least one ounce of steam distilled water daily for each pound of body weight thirty-two pounds, then thirty-two ounces of distilled water , one-hundred pounds of body weight, one-hundred ounces, etc.

In addition to the above de-worming procedures, some herbalists claim it is good to insert a peeled button of garlic into the rectum each night, six days a week, rest one day and repeat six days a week for several months, or give crushed garlic enemas. This will strengthen the bowel area, cut infections down, aid hemorrhoid area, and assist in discouraging worms. Keep the bowel area clean always if you want a healthy happy patient.

APPENDIX A

Bowel Cleansing and Nourishing

The following is the text of *Rejuvenation Through Elimination* by Dr. John R. Christopher now published (revised and expanded) as *Dr. Christopher s Guide to Colon Health.*

Our bodies must be kept clean, inside and out, to perform their tasks efficiently and smoothly. The body is the housing of the spirit, the operating force of life. With the spirit commanding a good clean structure smoother , happier lives will result. We have been told scripturally that our body is a temple, or tabernacle of God, and God will not dwell in an unclean tabernacle. So we must keep our bodies clean and in good repair for them to be comfortable abodes.

As we stand in small close areas with other people, their body odors can tell us a lot about their internal condition. The strong odor or fumes from alcoholic beverages emanate from the body and can be very repulsive. A constipated person also has a hard time covering his or her offensive body odor and uses deodorants and perfumes to disguise this unsavory condition.

We can compare this bad body odor caused by constipation to opening the door to our home after an extended absence and being greeted by the staggering foul odor of a backed up sewer. There are two ways this nauseating odor can be eliminated. One way is to cover the effect by buying room fresheners and spraying the area to neutralize the disagreeable scent. Reoccurrence is assured and the stench will return because this is only a temporary fix, nothing has been done about the cause of the smell. The wiser way is to remove the cause by unplugging and cleaning out the sewer line so there will be no more backing up of sewage.

Many of us have a sewage line that is backed up or constipated, and the horrible odor of halitosis comes out our front door (the mouth) as it is opened. Someone says, Y our breath is horrible, so most of us work on just the effect by popping in a mint or running for the mouthwash to cover our bad breath. If someone says, Whew you need a bath; the smell of your body is awful, most of us again work only on the effect and use underarm deodorant, perfumes, colognes, etc. We never think of cleaning up the cause, which not only affects how we smell, but our health.

Well over ninety percent of all disease comes from an unclean body whose sewer is backed up. A backed-up sewer means our filth has accumulated throughout the body. When this happens, you are dirty and filthy inside, the body does not operate as well, and mental processes often dwell on lower thoughts and ideas rather than on a higher plane.

Our human mechanism is like a car loaded with carbon and sludge, the timing is off, the electrical system is shorting, and is badly in need of a tune-up and overhaul. By grinding the valves, cleaning out the sludge in the oil system, tuning up the poorly functioning parts of the car, it will again run as good as new. Cleaning out our vehicles (our bodies) and getting a tune-up is the most important thing we can do to have a smoothly operating body that will use less fuel (food) and get better mileage and performance.

For this to happen we need to look at the bowel. Our bowels are the most neglected and ignored parts of our bodies. We need to know how this eliminative organ works so the large intestines can be kept clean and operate as desired and intended by the original creator of our bodies.

Inherent weaknesses are often handed down from generation to generation and it is our job to rebuild, renew and improve the (dietary and lifestyle) sins of our parents and pass on better habits to future generations. Because of improper eating and not taking care of our bodies, these weaknesses get handed down to our posterity. These could be sins of omission or sins of commission. Let s change the tide and build a better body so our offspring and the generations to come will become a stronger, happier and a more peaceful race of people.

Never will we have peace as long as we have constipated warriors sitting around the peace table glaring in hate at each other. Peace will come from clean, sweet, happy bodies and those who teach this natural lifestyle to their families through their example. These teachings can eventually spread worldwide.

The first steps to having a smooth-running, happy, efficient body is to first give it a three day juice cleanse and then start the mucusless diet as explained in *Dr. Christopher s Three Day Cleansing Program, Mucusless Diet, and Herbal Combinations*. This will start working on the cause of the malfunctions in the body, renewing the flesh and rebuilding organs. By continuing with this program, you are guaranteed to not have the problems of constipation and ill health any more during your life.

As we proceed along the line of the mucusless diet, do not panic for fear that you will starve. You will eat less, but you will have more vitality, less sickness, and your natural weight will be attained.

A good meal of a baked potato (if grown organically eat skin and all) or a steamed one with vegetable or olive oil, coarse freshly ground pepper and, if desired, chives and/or other condiment herbs for enhancing the flavor, along with a large vegetable salad, some steamed or low heated vegetables, fresh vegetable juice, a casserole of pre-soaked, low heated grains as a base (described in the above mentioned booklet see also *Regenerative Diet* by Dr. Christopher and *Transfiguration Diet*) and you will be satisfied, without that uncomfortable bloat or hidden hunger. You will be satisfied with less food without sluggishness. With this type of diet, you will eat approximately one-third of what you eat now, have more pep and energy, as well as free, easy bowel movements. This will not happen the first day but with the help of herbal aids to tone up the bowel area plus the diet and additional items we will tell you about, you will find new life!

A must for good health is to slow down the eating procedure. Relax and be happy while you eat. Discuss pleasant things during mealtime. Laugh a little and remember the old adage of a crust of bread with love is better than a banquet in contention. Chew each mouthful thoroughly, whether juice or solid food. Saliva is the key that opens the door to digestion. Without saliva mixed thoroughly with food or juice, the material goes down to the stomach and does not aid the gastric juices as Nature intended, causing much of the meal to be eliminated without proper assimilation.

What We Digest, Absorb, and Assimilate

Without cleanliness and tone in the entire alimentary tract, including the intestines, even the best of organic and regenerative-type foods may end up as waste and toxic ferment instead of readily-assimilable and life-giving elements absorbed by the blood-stream. Before life-properties in raw foods can reach the proper solution for absorption into the circulatory system, they must be successfully processed through three important digestive areas or mixing bowls. When any one of these areas is malfunctioning or is not properly utilized there is degenerative trouble. For, as Deschauer wisely asserted, W e live, not by what we eat, but by what we digest and absorb and assimilate.

The first digestive mixing bowl is the mouth, the teeth and the salivary glands. Here, the raw organic structures are, or should be, ground up fine with the teeth used as grinders and mixed well with the alkaline juices of saliva that are so necessary for preparing the starches for body use.

The body s three pairs of salivary glands are the parotid glands, (the largest), located in front of and below the ear, the ducts of which open into the mouth through the cheek just opposite the second molar teeth of the upper jaw; the submaxillary glands, which are about the size of a walnut and are located on each side beneath the lower jaw, their ducts opening into the mouth just under the tip of the tongue; and the sublingual glands located in the floor of the mouth, forming small ridges between the tongue and the gums of the lower jaw, having many ducts (some of which connect with the submaxillary glands). There are some one to two pints of saliva secreted daily into the mouth, containing, among other things, the important digestive ferment, ptyalin, which converts starches into grape sugar. Ptyalin s alkaline action is important in neutralizing acids, and it moistens and softens the food for passage through the esophagus.

The rate of secretion depends upon what is in the mouth, and although a button will stimulate it, there are certain savory and non-savory agents called sialogogues which will stimulate a ready flow of salivary juices. (Some herbal sialogogues include, betel leaves, blue flag root, cayenne, European elder bark, false sweet flag root, ginger root, hydrangea root, jaborandi root, and snake root.)

When food is swallowed it passes by the peristaltic action of the esophagus into the second digestive mixing bowl, where the gastric juices of hydrochloric acid, pepsin, are added. These dissolve the proteins and form food into a semifluid substance called chyme. The stomach is capable of considerable detention and the motions of its muscular action serve to knead and mix the gastric juices with the processing food. It has been estimated that there are some ten to twenty pints of gastric juices secreted during a twenty-four hour period. These juices restrict the action of saliva upon the starches while in the stomach, and also the fats are little affected thereby. The stomach normally completes its digestive action and is emptied of its contents every four to five hours.

Those agents that are specific aids in giving strength and tone to the stomach are called stomachics (herbs such as: agrimony, allspice, angelica, avens, bay leaves, betel leaves, thistle, camomile, caraway seed, cardamon seed, cascarilla, condurango, coriander, dandelion root, fennel seed, gentian, horsemint, lovage, nutmeg, peppermint, pimento, quassia, sweet flag, true unicorn, turkey rhubarb, and white cedar leaves). As the food is liquefied during the digestive processing by the stomach into chyme, gradually, in a very few minutes, this semi-fluid mass is expelled through the pylorus into the duodenum.

Almost immediately upon entering the duodenum, the chyme becomes mingled with pancreatic juices and bile. The pancreas is a compound secretory-excretory gland, taking elements from the blood and manufacturing a substance needed in the body, while the excretory gland separates elements from the blood for elimination from the body. The pancreas is situated behind the stomach, with its head at the curve of the duodenum. The bile is a golden-green fluid secreted by the liver. The liver weighs some sixty ounces (the largest gland in the body) and lies under the diaphragm and over the right kidney, upper portion of the ascending colon, and the pyloric end of the stomach.

During digestion in the intestines, both the bile and the pancreatic juices enter the duodenum about three inches below the pyloric valve through the common bile duct. When digestion is in progress, the duct carries the bile into the gall bladder, which is pear shaped and lodged in the tissue on the underside of the liver. When the duct becomes obstructed, the bile is absorbed into the blood and gives rise to a jaundiced condition in the tissues of the body. The bile is an alkaline agent which aids pancreatic juices in digestion, prevents fermentation in the intestines and stimulates the peristaltic action.

The healing agents that strengthen, tone and act upon the secretive functions of the liver are hepatic tonics (herbs such as: barberry, balimony, culver s root, dandelion, liverwort, Indian apple root, mandrake, marsh watercress, wahoo, wild yam, and wormwood). Agents that promote the flow of bile, by contracting the bile ducts, but not necessarily influencing or increasing the secretion of bile, are called cholagogues (herbs such as aloe gum, butternut bark, culver s root, and wahoo bark).

When this third mixing is completed, the vital and regenerative elements are ready to be absorbed into the blood through some ten million glands or rootlets which take three life-giving materials into the bloodstream, much like the root systems of plants assimilate necessary elements from the soil. Dr. Nowell clearly describes this digestive function and action which takes place within the intestinal tract, as follows:

> Both the large and small intestines consist of four coats similar to the stomach. The mucous membrane forming the inner surface of the small intestine has many small folds named Valvulae Connivents. These folds increase the area of the secreting surface. They also prevent food from passing too quickly through the intestines, thereby allowing full opportunity for the digestive juices to do their work.
>
> The inner surface of the small intestine is covered with a multitude of fine hairlike tubes called villi. These villi absorb notorious matter from the food in the intestinal tract.
>
> The mucous coat for both the large and small intestines is well supplied with glands. The glands vary. Some are tubular, some are globular (Peyer s Glands), some of these are single, others are in groups (Peyer s patches.) There are also others called Brunner s glands. These glands pour secretion

into the intestine. In view of the many villi and glands, the student will realize how necessary it is to keep the alimentary canal clean, that the value of the food may be conveyed to the bloodstream. It is undoubtedly true that by far the greatest majority of people seeking help when sick have allowed the intestinal tract to become clogged. This will upset the whole of the organism in one form or another.

Dr. Nowell goes on with his description of the digestive process:

From what has been said, it well be evident that the process of digestion continues through the small intestines. It does not, however, end there. The food passes through the small intestines into the large intestine through the cecum. The cecum becomes filled, the ileocecal valve closes and the walls of the cecum contract forcing the food into the ascending colon. The motions of the intestines are called peristaltic. They are wavelike. A peculiar feature of the motions of the ascending colon is that they are called antiperistaltic. This is because they pass both ways, i.e. away from the small intestines and toward them. This keeps the food moving back and forth and delays its passage. This gives time for the absorption of materials from the food.

Owing to the absorption of soluble materials from the food in its passage through the intestines, it becomes more solid or firm, until it becomes a mass suitable for ejection. This matter is called feces.

Feces consist of undigested foods, products of decomposition, bile, and other secretions. The color of the feces is primarily caused by the pigments from the bile. In jaundice, the stools are a light, clay color, showing that the bile is not flowing.

Defecation is the name given to the ejection of feces from the anus. The anus is the outer end of the rectum. Two strong muscles guard the anal canal the inner and outer sphincter muscles. The rectum is empty until just before defecation. Nerve stimuli produces peristaltic action in the colon using a small quantity of feces to enter the rectum. This arouses sensory nerves which bring about the desire to defecate. The rectum should be empty under normal conditions until just previous to defecation.

It is unwise to put off defecation when once the desire has arisen. The small portion of feces which enter the rectum bringing the desire to defecate will, when held there, become harder. Moreover, the presence of this in the rectum causes a dulling of the sensory nerves, thereby blunting the desire to defecate. This no doubt has much to do with causing constipation in many cases. Always respond to the call of nature as soon as possible.

With an understanding of our digestion and elimination, we can focus on correcting our weaknesses by learning how to cleanse out the old fecal matter that has been accumulating and gluing itself to the bowels and overall system of the body.

The Lower Bowel Formula (Fen-LB)

The injection and enema are useful for healing conditions such as piles, hemorrhoids, colitis, etc., and for cleaning putrid congestions from the intestinal tract, as in diarrhea and dysentery. Suppose you have a case of diarrhea the majority of people want a remedy that will stop it right away. But diarrhea is simply a condition in which the intestinal tract has become badly clogged that all the fecal solids are being held back and only the eliminative liquids are getting through. Would you believe it possible for people to have filth in them four, five, and ten or more years? It is a fact; we have seen with our own eyes.

The impurities accumulate with improper diet and life-style. When our bodies make an increase effort to clean that wastage out, the dirty channel, or intestinal tract, holds back large materials similar to the way overgrowth and trash can dam an irrigation ditch. When this happens, do not try to stop diarrhea, for it is simply the elimination of waste material, but use the appropriate means to remove the obstructing matter and clean the bowel out. The only exception to this rule should be when a person is too weak and the diarrhea is too heavy, wherein the diarrhea is stopped with agents such as red raspberry leaves, fresh peaches, or dried sunflower leaves, then a mild laxative is given, followed by other agents that will gently remove the obstruction and build up the area again.

You will be surprised at how much filth three quarts of a stimulating injection will expel. However, injections or enemas are really not the permanent solution for this problem, as they only relieve the problem temporarily, and the peristaltic muscles do not work when enemas are being used for eliminative purposes. Enemas are only a crutch in solving the problem. What is needed here is The Lower Bowel Formula, which is a corrective food for the intestinal tract.

In bowel movements, no two people are alike. Often we start the Lower Bowel Formula one capsule three times daily, then reduce to a single capsule a day. When the formula gets to the outside walls of the intestine and breaks loose some of this hard fecal matter, this old matter will go down the intestines and begin to clog up the tract.

So during your cleansing cycles when the body is throwing off more of its accumulated wastage, or when the Lower Bowel Formula is getting to the outside of the intestinal tract and breaking loose some of the hard fecal matter from the walls remember to accentuate or intensify your use of the Lower Bowel Formula and take the necessary quantity up to maybe even twenty capsules a day to break it loose. When this is accomplished, reduce your dosage.

If you discover undigested food in the fecal matter, this generally means that the bowel is so badly clogged that food is going through the tract without proper assimilation. In addition, when bloating of the bowels occurs, this is a signal to get back on to another cleanse (see Appendix B). A condition of sciatic rheumatism will always develop where the sigmoid (end) portion of the lower bowel becomes congested, and the toxic poisons from the bowel subsequently flow into the adjacent area, irritating the nerves controlling the sacroiliac and, in turn, throwing it out of place and so goes the vicious cycle!

A periodic purification and cleansing of the lower intestinal tract is very important for us. This is your sewage system and when the eliminative function is efficient and clean, you do not have to worry about sluggishness or toxification in the system.

Cleansing The Bowel For Greater Vitality

What is the source of intestinal complaints? When we eat unwholesome food, a certain amount of its mucous forming substance stays in the intestine by adhering to the walls. This mucus glues itself on like wallpaper paste and forms layers around the intestinal walls. As each additional layer forms through incorrect eating habits, the muscular and absorptive tissues become thickly covered and proportionately less functional. As these fecal layers become hardened and continue to grow thicker, eventually only a small hole will remain in the center of the lower bowel. So the matter of fecal elimination is entirely deceptive when we do not sufficient understanding of the correct and normal bowel function.

We often say, I have bowel movements every day. Sure, we have bowel movements every day, but what really happens is our old fecal matter encrusted on our intestinal walls prevents the food from being assimilated. Instead of assimilating the nutrition from undigested food, we utilize only ten percent of its real value, and the rest is wasted on down the eliminative drain. With the intestinal tract so badly layered and clogged, your food simply cannot get through to the absorptive villi and functional tissues on the walls. The result is a weakened bowel that loses its elasticity and balloons out.

These hardened layers in the bowels are just like rings in a tree, which multiply during each year and vary according to the habits and types of materials consumed. When a person suffers from halitosis or bad breath, this is nature s way of saying, You have a toxic bowel condition.

One patient asked, Why is it that I only eat one-fifth of what I used to eat, and when I was eating five times as much I had a bowel movement every day, and I thought that was adequate. But now that I am eating only one-fifth of what I formerly ate, I am having from five to seven bowel movements each and every day and they are massive ones, and I am eating less! You figure that one out, will you?

Well, when I was a boy and working in a cabinet shop, we had an old glue pot. The inside of the pot, as the years rolled on, got smaller and smaller due to the glue adhering to the inside. Because it was a very expensive glue pot, we could not use the hammer on it to break the substance loose, so we had to reverse the process we had to soak it out! The same is true with the human colon, we have to soak out the old fecal matter to strengthen our colon.

The abnormal intestinal condition that is found among most people today is from improper eating habits that accumulate waste upon the intestinal walls. This waste becomes dehydrated and compacted like dried fruit, dried flax, etc., and it starts to swell when water gets into it, creating a ballooned pocket in our intestinal tract. A mucus condition in the colon is generally food that gets caught and rots in these pockets, which enemas cannot touch.

Ridding the body of poison is most important, and animal products are the most mucus-forming. We have thirty-two feet of intestinal tract, and when we plug it up with meat, cheese, milk, etc., the waste materials remain too long and the uric acid passes through and toxifies our whole system.

What happens when congestion occurs in the intestines while you are on the Cleansing Program? In one day, with the help of the Lower Bowel herbs, you may soak loose what has been accumulating there during at least a three week layering period of some previous time. The closer the cleansing process approaches the intestinal walls, the harder the encrusted fecal matter is. It is often broken off and comes out in pieces just like an old plastic or rubber hose! A frequent swelling in the abdomen results during the cleanse as the Lower Bowel agents begin soaking through. However, when this filth is cleaned out, you will feel like a million dollars revitalized and young again.

For instance, in one case we had a boy who for eight months was having somewhat regular and normal bowel movements, then one evening he called his father in the night and was amazed that he had dropped a five pound load--he completely filled the toilet! What had happened was that accumulations from years back had finally broken loose. When this cleansing process is completed, the food value finally returns to the outside intestinal wall, the tissues are fed properly and the peristaltic muscles once again start working.

Now this is where our Lower Bowel Formula wins, because it is not a crutch. It cleans the liver, the gall bladder, starts the bowel flowing, and stimulates the peristaltic muscles to begin working and kneading out waste. You can take colonics, irrigations, enemas, or herbal laxatives until they are running out your ears, but as long as the peristaltic muscles are not functioning, no permanent healing can be accomplished. So remember, as long as you have a polluted and congested bowel, you are getting only about ten percent of your food value, and your body degenerates as long as this persists.

What are the benefits of a cleansed and properly functioning bowel? The patient mentioned previously who is eating only one-fifth of his former quantity of food now has more strength, more endurance, more pep and energy than he ever had, and he is happier! But these are not the only advantages, especially for those planning to survive the troubled days ahead; for when you become more efficient with your food assimilation within the body, then you will be able to go three to four times as long on the same quantity of food as the average individual. Thus, you will not need as much food to survive during critical times, a regular two year food supply is going to last you eight or nine years. As you clean out and tone up the bowel, you will be assured a greater nutritional efficiency for the entire body system, and all the other glands and organs will be properly fed and regenerated! When your body is cleansed, you will also be able to assimilate various types of foods and get the food value out of them that nobody else can.

For the first thirty-five years of my life, I had to have three immense meals a day and piece in between to get through an eight hour work period. Now, it is many a day that I will be up at five o clock in the morning, and not eat until two or three o clock in the afternoon. My second meal will be between midnight and one o clock in the morning, and these will both be small meals, as the first one will be a salad and the second one will be some healthy Chinese food. However, I am doing eighteen to twenty hours on that much food, when I could not have done that before not even in an eight hour day!

Men and women repeatedly raise their hands in our herb classes and volunteer such testimonials, as Since we have been on this Cleansing Program, we have cut our food bill straight in half!
The following is from *Colon Hygiene* by John Harvey Kellogg, M.D.:

Exercise. Bodily activity is another way of mechanically stimulating the intestine. Vigorous exercise sets the diaphragm and abdominal muscles at work in such a way that the intestines are, between the two, vigorously kneaded and squeezed and thus stimulated into action.

Every farmer knows the constipating effect of idleness upon his horses and cattle. Most observing persons have noted in their own experience the advantage of taking a brisk walk before or after breakfast.

The sedentary man or woman not only loses the immediate effect which results from the increased activity of the diaphragm and abdominal muscles, but his abdominal muscles become permanently weakened, relaxed, lacking in tone, and incapable of supporting the intestines in their proper place, thus adding a number of other factors which contribute very materially to the lessening of intestinal activity.

Posture. A stooped or relaxed posture when sitting or standing tends strongly to induce constipation by weakening the abdominal muscles and causing congestion of the liver and all other abdominal organs. The viscera, overfilled with blood, and lacking the support of the abdominal muscles, becomes prolapsed. The colon falls with the rest; the intestinal contents stagnate; the bowel becomes distended; the ileocecal valve becomes incompetent; infection travels up the small intestine, and a long list of ills result.

An erect posture secures proper exercise of the muscles of the trunk, correct breathing, normal circulation of blood in the viscera, and promotes in a high degree normal bowel movement.

A further cause of injury is the lowering of the diaphragm and diminished action of this important muscle, which when normally active applies to the colon and other active viscera a sort of rhythmic massage which is a valuable aid to bowel action.

Influences which lessen intestinal movements. There are certain foods and other agents that produce a decided slowing influence upon intestinal movements, either directly or indirectly, through the suppression of the normal stimuli. Liquid foods, such as soups, gruels, porridges, and purees contain so little solid matter that the bulk, considerable though it may be when the food is eaten, is soon reduced to a very small volume. On this account, liquid foods are almost always constipating. The only exceptions are those liquid foods which contain much sugar, acids or fats.

Pasty cereals such as oatmeal are decidedly constipating in their influence because of their pasty consistency and the little mastication which they generally receive. New bread, hot biscuits, noodles, and doughy foods of all sorts are likewise objectionable.

Fruit juices of all sorts are most suitable for almost all forms of sickness. They contain choice nutrients in a form needing no digestion, ready for immediate absorption and assimilation.

Orange juice or freshly pressed juice of apples, grape, or other sweet or sub-acid fruit, is ideal nourishment for the sick. In the absence of these fresh fruits, dried fruit soaked long in distilled water may furnish a very fair substitute.

Colon disease. It is probable that more disease, premature old age and death, misery and even crime originate from constipation than from any other bodily disorder. Constipation is not of itself a disease but a symptom, the cause of which may be disease or simply neglect.

There are several very prevalent errors respecting the colon and its functions which are probably responsible for most of the mischief which arises from disorders of this part of the body.

One of the most universal and mischievous of errors about the humble colon is that its function is one which modesty imperatively demands shall be concealed even at the expense of great suffering. Although recent times have given us a greater abundance of restroom facilities, many public places such as grocery stores, malls and shopping plazas, banks and etc., still do not offer adequate facilities either for patrons or passersby. And many of these establishments do not allow use of the restrooms to non-patrons. Such conditions help promote the standard norm of holding it, which is the beginning of bowel dysfunction.

Another modern problem is that in today s fast paced society it has become an inconvenience to take time out to allow the body to cleanse itself and then continue on. There are even accounts from natural healers who have worked with people who had a bowel movement once a month, and even once every other month! This was because of the modern working life-styles that could not allow a few minutes each day to go to the restroom.

Unfortunately, as we have become more civilized, we have begun to put industry before regularity. Most jobs, and many public schools, do not offer access to restrooms when needed, and the employee or student must postpone their body s desired function to suit the demand of business or convenience.

The results are most disastrous. The majority of chronic human ills are the results of this neglect.

Another common error which is held by most medical men, as well as by the laity, is that the stool should be formed. This is a false notion that has grown out of the constipation habit which prevails among civilized folk.

The vegetarian Hindus of Armistar, who live chiefly on ground wheat and vegetables, according to Dr. A. H. Browne, have lar ge, bulky, and not formed, but pultaceous stools.

A well-formed stool always means constipation. The significance is that the colon is packed full like a sausage and that the fecal matters have been so long retained that they have been compacted by the absorption of water. The whole colon is filled, and the bowel movement is the result of the pressure of the incoming food residues at the other end. When the body s wastes are promptly discharged as they should be, the colon never contains the residues of more than two meals and at the after-breakfast movement should be completely emptied so that the disinfecting and lubricating mucus which its walls secrete may have its opportunity to cleanse and disinfect the body s garbage receptacle, and thus keep it in a sanitary condition.

The California doctor who advised his patient to restrain his desire for a bowel movement at night and hold it until the next morning so that he might have a well-formed stool, had not the first conception of the normal function of the colon.

The idea that one bowel movement a day is normal and efficient evacuation of the bowels is another error which is universally entertained. One bowel movement a day is a positive indication of constipation. X-ray examinations of the colon after a test meal show that, in persons whose bowels move once a day, the body wastes are usually retained for fifty hours or more. Hurst, of London, and many other authorities finding this condition almost universal have been led to regard it as normal, but in this, they are certainly in error. X-ray examinations show that in eight hours from the beginning of a meal the process of digestion has been completed, the digested food has been absorbed, and the unusable residue has been pushed half way through the colon, and is within two and a half feet of the lower opening of the colon. In eight hours the food has travelled more than twenty-five feet or ten times the distance which remains to be travelled. The work of digestion is finished, the useful part of the food has been absorbed, there remains nothing to be done but to dispose of the indigestible and useless residue by pushing it along two or three feet further. Certainly, no good reason can be assigned for the further retention of the waste matters. It is indeed highly absurd to suppose that forty hours are needed to transport the feces two and a half feet when they have already travelled twenty-five feet in eight hours.

The bowels should move at least three times a day or

after each meal. Four movements daily is a still better rhythm and is easily established by a biological regimen, as this the writer has proven in many exceptional cases involving thousands of patients who have been willing to take the time to train their bowels by the means of a proper diet and other simple and natural means.

Putrefaction. The carmine capsule test shows that in most cases in which the bowels move once daily, the waste disposal function is always several days in arrears. The colon contains the waste and residues of several meals anywhere from five to twenty or even more so that there is ample opportunity for the putrefactive process to get well under way.

Putrefaction is the source of the foul odor and gases which originate in the colon, and which are not only most offensive to the sense of smell, but as is well known, are also highly poisonous, and may give rise to nausea, biliousness, loss of appetite, bad breath, dingy skin, headache, Bright s disease, and a host of other grave disorders.

Hasty eating. Insufficient mastication is a fault peculiar to civilized men. The savage, as well as the monkey and all lower animals that are provided with teeth for grinding food, masticates his food with the greatest thoroughness. A skull in the writer s possession shows the teeth of an ancient mound builder, a Malkelkos Indian. The well-worn appearance of the teeth affords sufficient evidence of the thoroughness with which they were used to grind the nuts and cereal foods eaten by ancient Indians.

Meat eating. Carnivorous animals have a short alimentary canal and a smooth colon. The movement of food-stuffs along this short, smooth passage is rapid. This is necessary for the preservation of the life of the animal, as undigested remnants of meat long retained in the body necessarily undergo putrefactive changes with the production of ptomaines and poisons. The digestion of meat leaves little residue, hence a person who lives chiefly on meat suffers from constipation, a condition which favors the putrefaction of undigested food remnants, and this, by creating an acidic condition of the intestines, paralyzes the bowel and further increases the constipation.

Meat also causes constipation through the fact that it encourages putrefaction of the colon both by introducing putrefactive organisms in great numbers and by providing material which is best calculated to encourage the growth of putrefactive organisms in the colon. Through the putrefaction of undigested remnants of the meat eaten, ammonia and other substances are formed which paralyze the bowel.

The infection of the bowel which results from meat-eating also gives rise to colitis and causes a spastic or contracted condition of the descending colon, a condition found in the most obstinate forms of constipation.

Insufficient fluid. Most persons who suffer from constipation habitually drink too little water. It is difficult to account for this scanty use of a necessity of life, which costs little and is of such inestimable value to the body. Water is far more immediately necessary for the support of life than is food. A man may live six to eight weeks without tasting food in any form, but ten days at the most is the limit of human life without water. The consequence of a scanty use of water is abnormal dryness of the feces, which delays their passage through the lower colon, and often causes an actual stoppage in the pelvic colon or the rectum.

Persons who sweat much, either as the result of hot weather, vigorous exercise, or hot baths, are likely to suffer from constipation, unless special care is taken to supply the body with water sufficient to make good the loss. The skin ordinarily throws off as perspiration an ounce and a half of water each hour, or more than a quart in twenty-four hours. By active exercise or sweating baths, this amount may be increased to thirty or forty ounces in an hour. The kidneys excrete two to three pints daily. It is evident, therefore, that care must be exercised to replace the water that is lost through the skin and the kidneys.

In diabetes, there is a great loss of water through the kidneys. This, also, must be made up by drinking wholesome liquids. If these losses are not made good, the thirsty tissues will absorb as much water as possible from the feces, thus causing hardening and retention in the lower bowel.

Scanty and highly colored urine is an evidence that the tissues are in need of water. Dryness of the skin often testifies to the same need.

Water should be taken in proper quantity irrespective of thirst. It may be made palatable by the addition of fresh fruit juices, especially fresh lemon juice.

For the average person a good plan is to take a couple of glasses of water on rising, and the same amount before retiring at night. A glassful should be taken half an hour before dinner and supper, and an equal amount two hours after eating. The free use of oranges or orange juice, and of other juicy fruits, serves the same purpose as water drinking, to the extent of the liquid which they supply.

Persons suffering from obesity or diabetes are sometimes restricted in the drinking of water, with the result that constipation is produced, if this condition does not already exist. This should never be done.

In all cases in which there is a tendency to dryness of the stools, water should be taken in increased quantity. It is also important in such cases, also, to diminish the amount of salt eaten. The addition of salt to the food creates thirst for water to dissolve it and to aid in its elimination through the skin and the kidneys.

Children, as well as adults, need much more water than they are usually given. Meat eaters and those who use salt freely require a much larger amount of water than do those who adhere to a low protein diet and who use little salt.

Exercise. The excellent effects that walking has upon bowel activity are well known. Riding is also of great advantage in the same way. These exercises, and many others, mechanically stimulate the colon as well as all parts of the intestinal tract by communicating to it a continued series of slight shocks, by which reflex movements are excited. The active play of children is as necessary to maintain proper bowel action as for muscular development. The movements of skipping, hopping and jumping are especially useful because they induce sudden vigorous contractions of the abdominal muscles and vigorous diaphragm movements by which the colon is compressed and stimulated. The folk dancing of the Middle Ages, which has been revived in recent years, is to be highly commended as a health measure for the above reasons. It is important, however, to make a clear distinction between the varied and vigorous movements of the folk dance, in simple dress and under wholesome conditions, and the monotonous and restrained movements of the social dance, in full dress and under conditions always physically, and not infrequently morally unwholesome.

Those whose occupations are such as to give them plenty of exercise are fortunate in being able to lead lives which in large measure conform to natural requirements. Such persons never need suffer from constipation if they eat proper food, drink an abundance of water at least three to five pints daily and take care to give the bowels an opportunity for movement after each meal, and a prompt excavation whenever there is a call.

Those who are compelled to lead sedentary lives must take daily and regular exercise of a sort calculated to benefit the bowels if they would escape the evils of constipation and its sedentary results.

Exercises which combat constipation. The exercises that are of the greatest value in cases of constipation are those which bring into strong action the muscles of the abdomen. The abdominal muscles are generally weak and relaxed, and the intra-abdominal pressure is consequently low.

By appropriate exercises the weak muscles may be strengthened, the intra-abdominal pressure may be raised and the colon may be thus enabled to contract with sufficient impetus to expel its contents.

Hill climbing. Hill climbing is a more valuable exercise than walking on level ground because the abdominal muscles are brought into more active play. When mountain climbing is not an available form of exercise, nearly the same results may be obtained by climbing a ladder or by walking up and down stairs. The writer has also made use of the treadmill as the means of securing muscular exercise similar to that required in hill climbing.

Horseback riding. Horseback riding is especially indicated as an exercise for constipation. However, persons accustomed to riding must ride a considerable distance or ride a hard trotting horse for this to be an effective exercise.

Rowing. Rowing is one of the very best exercises to combat constipation, provided the chest is held high during the exercise, and especially if care is taken to give the trunk as strong a backward movement as possible. But one must avoid holding the trunk forward with the shoulders rounded and the chest depressed.

Tennis. Tennis is highly recommended for young persons and those who are sufficiently strong to engage in this form of exercise without injury. This very popular game is, however, too vigorous for persons with weak hearts.

The Medicine Ball. This is a capital exercise for persons who are sufficiently strong. It brings the muscles of the trunk into vigorous action.

Work exercises. The movements of chopping, digging, swinging the hammer and mowing are highly valuable exercises if taken with due care to maintain the body in an erect position. Many household occupations, such as scrubbing, washing, and general housework are excellent forms of exercise when the correct posture is maintained.

Posture exercises. Maintenance of an erect position of the trunk is of first importance of persons suffering from constipation. When the chest is lowered, as in sitting in a relaxed attitude, the distance between the breastbone and the pelvis is diminished so that the large muscles which form the front of the abdominal wall are shortened and relaxed. In this attitude, the muscles cannot be contracted sufficiently to produce the proper degree of intra-abdominal pressure. When the chest is held high, the rectus muscles are stretched, and are thus able by contraction to produce the maximum effect in compressing the colon. Flat-chested persons are predisposed to constipation because of inefficient action of the abdominal muscles.

The ordinary chair must be regarded to a very considerable degree as responsible for the prevalence of flat chest and round shoulders, and the evils which result from this deformity. It is possible to sit in an erect attitude in a chair of any shape, but with a chair with a straight back, a constant effort of forcible contraction of the muscles is required to maintain the body in an erect position. The moment the muscles are permitted to relax, the trunk falls into an abnormal and unhealthy attitude, the spinal column being curved backward instead of forward, as is natural and necessary for health.

As the results of an habitually wrong attitude in sitting, the same improper attitude is maintained when standing and walking, and the figure becomes deformed. A flat chest, round shoulders, and a forward carriage of the hips are characteristics to be found in the great majority of persons who lead sedentary lives, especially those who sit much at their work, such as accountants, writers, teachers, and professional people generally. One of the first things, then, for a constipated person to do is to correct his standing and sitting attitudes. This may be done by careful execution of the following exercises, which the writer has employed for more than 25 years with much satisfaction in the treatment of cases of this sort.

To correct the standing posture. Stand against a straight wall. Place heels, hips, shoulders, head and hands firmly against the wall. Now bend the head backwards as far as possible, or until the eyes look straight up to the ceiling, at the same time permitting the chest and shoulders to move forward. While holding the head in this position, press the hands firmly against the wall. Draw the chin down to position without allowing the shoulders to move backward, still holding the body rigid, allowing the arms to fall at the sides. In this position the chest will be held high and the abdominal muscles well drawn in. While holding this position, execute movements with the arms, raising them above the head in swimming movements, etc.

This is the correct standing position and should, as much as possible, be constantly maintained in standing and walking. It is impossible, of course, to hold the muscles constantly rigid. In relaxing, however, care should be taken to keep the chest forward, so that the body does not fall back into the former incorrect attitude.

Exercises to correct the sitting posture. When sitting upon a chair or stool, preferably the latter, proceed as follows:

Place the hands on the hips with the thumbs behind. Bend the head backwards so as to look straight up at the ceiling, then bend forward as far as possible while still keeping the eyes on the ceiling. Make firm pressure with the thumbs, and while pressing hard, bring the body up to the erect position. Still keeping the eyes upon the ceiling, holding the elbows back as far as possible, and without lessening the pressure of the thumbs, bring the chin down to position.

If this movement is executed according to directions, it will bring the body into perfect position, with the chest raised high and the abdominal muscles well drawn in.

Resisting the Call. The practice of resisting the call of Nature to discharge from the body its accumulated wastes and rubbish is almost universal among civilized people, as the result of a social refinement of manners and modesty which lead to the concealment of certain animalistic body functions. That this is the result of what is commonly called false modesty cannot be denied, and yet there are few that would desire that this false modesty should be altogether laid aside. It is important, however, that every person, children as well as adults, should at a very early age be fully instructed respecting the evil results or resisting Nature s call and thus thwarting one of the most important functions of the body.

The use of tobacco. Numerous laboratory experiments have shown that the use of tobacco in any form has a paralyzing effect upon the splanchnic nerves. Without the aid of these sympathetic nerves normal, rhythmical bowel movements are impossible. The fact that some persons observe an apparently favorable influence from smoking is accepted as evidence that the effects of the weed are favorable to the bowels. These cases are exceptional and misguided. In general, the use of tobacco is highly injurious to the intestine.

Alcohol and other narcotic drugs. Alcoholic beverages of all sorts tend to produce constipation by causing chronic intestinal catarrh, ulcer of the stomach, and paralysis of the sympathetic nerves.

We do not recommend laxatives such as purchased from a drug store, or herbal laxatives in many cases from health food stores that are just a laxative. These become habit forming. Instead, we recommend the use of herbs to feed and rebuild the bowel, to activate the dormant peristaltic muscles and clean off the bowel walls for complete assimilation of foods going through the intestinal tract.

Water and Juice

An abundant supply of wholesome unsweetened fruit and vegetable juice (especially raw spinach juice) should be used daily. In addition, drink plenty of distilled water to supply liquid to the body. The human body under normal circumstances is made up of approximately eighty percent fluid; this must be replenished daily in the form of liquid intake. Only the best of liquid should be used to replace the daily loss through elimination from urination, perspiration and from the bowel area, etc. The use of inorganic drinks and beverages high in sugar, synthetic sweetenings, chemical additives and artificial colorings (soft drinks), the use of alcoholic beverages and polluted stream or tap waters is as ridiculous as pouring salt, sugar or dirty water into the gas tank of your car.

N. W. Walker, D.Sc., has written an excellent book entitled *Fresh Vegetable and Fruit Juices*. In this book he says:

> When the food is raw, whether whole or in the form of juice, every atom in such food is vital organic. Therefore, the oxalic acid in our raw vegetables and their juices is organic, and is not only beneficial, but essential for physiological functions of the body.
>
> The oxalic acid in cooked and processed foods, however, is definitely dead, or inorganic, and as such is positively both pernicious and destructive. Oxalic acid readily combines with calcium. If these are both organic, the result is a beneficial constructive combination, as the former helps the digestive assimilation of the latter, at the same time stimulating the peristaltic functions of the body.
>
> When the oxalic acid becomes inorganic by cooking or processing the foods that contain it, then this acid forms an interlocking compound with the calcium, even combining with the calcium in other foods eaten during the same meal, destroy-

ing the nourishing value of both. This results in such a serious deficiency of calcium that it has even been known to cause decomposition of the bones (osteoporosis). This is the reason I never eat cooked or canned spinach.

As to the oxalic acid itself, when converted into an inorganic acid by cooking or processing the food, it often results in causing inorganic oxalic acid crystals to form in the kidneys.

It is worthy of notice that the minerals in our foods, iron, for example, frequently cannot be assimilated and used completely if they have become inorganic through cooking, and often prevent the utilizing of other elements through chemical and other action. Thus, the iron in fresh, raw spinach juice may be utilized 100%, but only one-fifth of that, or less, would be available in cooked spinach.

It is well to bear in mind, therefore, that as the organic oxalic acid is so vital to our well-being, the fresh raw juice of the vegetables containing it should be used daily to supplement the eating of these raw vegetables included in our daily salads.

The most abundant supply of organic oxalic acid is found in fresh raw spinach and rhubarb.

Aids in Elimination from Certain Foods

To assist in keeping the bowels clean, and feeding and nourishing them at the same time, add 1/4 or more flaxseed and/or psyllium seed to the whole, uncracked grains being prepared for breakfast or noonday meal as is explained on the low heating procedure in *Three Day Cleanse and Mucusless Diet* (see Appendix B) and *Transfiguration Diet*.

Laxative Gruel. If you desire additional assistance to the bowel, prepare flaxseed and/or psyllium seed, licorice root, marshmallow root, and comfrey root, each in three parts, and add one part lobelia herb. Sweeten with honey if desired. Use as little or as much as you require for assisting in free, easy bowel movements. The flaxseed and the psyllium seed give bulk; licorice root is a mild aperient (mildest of laxatives); marshmallow root is to assist clearance where hard stools are prevalent; comfrey root is the healer and rebuilder of weak areas and gives lubrication; and lobelia is the accentuating herb.

Confectionery Type Bowel Aid. Make these delicious candies using the following instructions as a basic guide and vary as you wish.

To each pint of chopped or ground up dried fruit (raisins, prunes, apricots, peaches, apples, dates, or figs), mix in one ounce powdered flaxseed, one ounce powdered licorice root, one ounce powdered slippery elm bark, and add enough sorghum or blackstrap molasses to mold it into small balls. Roll these in half powdered carob and half slippery elm bark so the confection is not sticky. Use these as needed. The ingredients and amounts can be adjusted as desired.

Fruits and Raw Vegetables. Use plenty of fresh, ripe fruit, or unsulphered dried fruit, lots of raw fibrous vegetables to chew on, or use in salads, and small amounts of whole bran the type supplied by the millers or from a health store. Add honey and water, or fresh fruit or vegetable juice to moisten the bran for easier eating. The person using plenty of whole uncracked low-heated grains doesn t need additional bran as a rule.

The test for wholesome live grains is that after presoaking and low-heating (under 140 degrees F), they are still alive and will grow. If you have some whole grain (wheat, buckwheat, rye, millet, barley, flaxseed) single or in your favorite combination left over after a meal, and/or some whole grain as a base used for a casserole, take some of these grains out and plant them in a row or furrow in the backyard. In another row, plant some Wheaties, granola and a loaf of bread, cover them, water and care for this new little garden and see which row will sprout and grow. The row that produces is the wholesome (Webster s unabridged dictionary defines wholesome as with the life therein as in its original state) food that is alive and will give life to your body . The row that remains dormant is dead and is only a filler without true life in it.

Exercise. As Kellogg mentioned, to assist in having natural bowel movements it is well to exercise. In all forms of exercise one should remember that the body areas firm up and strengthen themselves with exercise up to, that is until, the time of fatigue. Continuing on after fatigue, we lose value rapidly. Just before the time of tiring, stop and rest before continuing on and gradually exercising can become easy, and stamina will increase without fatigue or damage.

One of the best types of exercise is to walk with a long stride from the hips, increasing each day the length of time doing it, and find how enjoyable this will be. Swimming, dancing, and jogging are all beneficial if not overdone.

Herbal Aids. Over a period of time, the mucusless diet, with its plenty of whole grains, fibers from fruits and vegetables, nuts and seeds will regulate bowel excretion. However, with a buildup of layers of mucus linings as coatings on the bowel walls, it is best to use foods that are specific in toning, rebuilding and strengthening this area. These special foods are herbs, or the Lower Bowel Formula. For many years we have been recommending this combination of herbs, and it has done remarkable good for many thousands of people.

Here is the basic cleansing and rebuilding herbal formula. This combination has been formulated with the average individual in mind and meets nearly all general problem requirements. Consult a competent health practitioner for any uncommon health problems not found within the scope of this formula.

If the stool seems too loose when using the Lower Bowel Formula, then cut down; but if it is difficult to get a bowel movement and the stool is hard and takes a long time to eliminate, then increase the amount until the stools become soft and loosely-formed. In very difficult cases, you could take even up to forty of these capsules a day, since these herbs are only food and do no damage to you. After the hard material has broken loose and is eliminating more freely, the copious amounts of eliminating matter will gradually decrease (these are hard encrustations of fecal matter that have been stored in the bowel for many years that are breaking loose and soaking up intestinal liquids).

But do not reduce the Lower Bowel Formula dosage so much at this point that you lose the advantageous momentum and continuity of elimination. In most cases, the improper diet has caused the peristaltic muscles to quit working, and it will take six to nine months with the aid of the Lower Bowel Formula for the average individual to clean out the old fecal matter and rebuild the bowel structure sufficiently, and have these muscles work entirely on their own.

Most of us have pounds of old, dried fecal matter that is stored up in the colon and is toxifying the system and keeping the food from being assimilated, and because of this putrefied condition, we engorge ourselves with many times more than the actual body requirements. In the process we wear out our bodies in trying to get sufficient food value and are still always hungry and eating. Whereas after the bowel is cleansed, the food is readily assimilated and the person can sustain himself on about one-third the quantity of his current food consumption at some four or five times increase in more power, energy, vitality and life.

The clean body is able to assimilate the simple food values through the cell structures in the colon instead of being trapped in a maze of wastage and inhibited by the hard fecal casing on the intestinal walls where the largest part of the nutritional substance becomes pushed on and eliminated before it can do any good. When the body is completely clean, the Lower Bowel Formula will no longer be necessary then your food will be your medicine and your medicine will be your food. Once the bowel is cleansed, this Lower Bowel Formula should only be used as needed, providing you have stayed on the program properly. Each herb in this formula is explained here in detail.

Barberry

If this is not available you may substitute Oregon Grape root, also called Rocky Mountain Grape root, which is the same family and will do the same type of job. This family of herbs acts as a specific for the liver and gall bladder (hepatic) area causing the bile to flow freely instead of being congealed and sluggish, and this bile acts as a mild laxative. The herb is also alterative (blood purifying), antisyphilitic, and tonic.

Cayenne

Cayenne is slightly laxative, stimulates the organs as it passes through, aids in rebuilding varicose conditions, and eliminating cholesterol from the area. It does a real cleaning and rebuilding job.

Cascara Sagrada

This herb is called sacred bark and in small amounts, as used here, is a mild laxative. It is also a tonic for the peristaltic muscles, increasing the secretions of the stomach, liver and pancreas, and is very remarkable in its action in torpor of the colon and constipation. It is, unquestionably, one of the very best and safest laxatives ever discovered.

Ginger

Its common name is Jamaica ginger. This herb is excellent for correcting flatulence (gas in the stomach). We need this herb to alleviate gas that is accumulated as the bile starts flowing into this area, mixing with old fecal matter and forming this condition. It is also an aid for relieving cramps and pains.

Goldenseal

This wonderful herb is a tonic, mild laxative, alterative (for mucus membranes), detergent, antiseptic and anti-emetic. This is a healer and kills infection, a blood purifier and aperient (mild laxative).

Lobelia

This is the accentuating herb that makes any formula work more smoothly and more efficiently. It is also an anti-spasmodic, a nervine, and will assist in cases of cramps and painful conditions.

Red Raspberry Leaves

Herein is an herb that assists in supplying iron to the system in the form of citrate of iron. Upon this compound depends the remarkable blood making and regulating properties as well as the astringent and contracting action on the internal tissues and membranes. This herb is also hemostatic, antiseptic and anti-diarrhea.

Turkey Rhubarb Root

Turkey (or China) rhubarb is such a mild aperient (laxative) that it can be used for tiny babies because it gives smooth, easy, no-cramping bowel movements. This herb has such a complex makeup. It is a laxative, astringent, tonic, stomachic, brisk purgative and valuable in effecting a quick, safe emptying of the bowels. It does not clog or produce an after-constipation as so many cathartics do. It is especially useful in diarrhea caused by irritating substances in the intestines. It not only removes these substances, but its delayed astringent action checks the diarrhea.

Fennel

This herb is noted for its relief in flatulency (gas) indigestion, cramps and spasms, nausea, pinworms, and in hepatic conditions (liver, gall bladder malfunctions).

Each of these nine herbs have a specific job to do and combined they make an herbal food for the bowel (small and large) area. Because we have accumulated filth and fecal matter in our bowels for often many years, using this formula for nine months to a year or more in some cases is not severe at all. Working with both the mucusless diet and the Lower Bowel Formula, you can have continually easy bowel movements for the rest of your life. And if you continually observe the mucusless diet, soon no Lower Bowel Formula will be needed.

Remember, this herbal combination is not habit forming or one that you have to increase as time goes on, but one that works on the cause and not just as a laxative or flush for temporary relief. You can watch the amount of this Lower Bowel Formula and regulate it and eventually reduce it until you have easy, regular bowel movements without the use of this aid at all. Your proper diet will help sustain regular movements.

The formulas that we are using in our programs are those that have been tried and proven over the many years of our research and practice. There are compatible formulas available that we use. The Lower Bowel Formula is food for the bowel and an assistant to the organs, designed to clean and rebuild. As with any reconstruction program, all procedures should be done with thought and care. Health does not happen overnight, but over a period of months.

During the first years of the Lower Bowel Formula s use, during the 1940s, people said that it was griping. For this reason, we added the ginger. Some asked, Why not add an aid in the combination for the nausea that happened in a few cases? So we added red raspberry leaves to relieve this condition and to add lost iron and fruit acids that were causing this problem. This was an additional help to each user as well as to the ones who were upset. In all our formulas, as well as in these cases, each herb has its own specific job to do.

Remember the important function of your bowel and give it the consistent nourishment and care it requires to keep the body clean and healthy. Constipation is the root of all dis-ease, therefore let us take the time to exercise, correct our posture, drink plenty of distilled water and fresh juices, and eat wholesome, living foods that will aid our bowels to serve us more perfectly.

APPENDIX B

THE THREE-DAY CLEANSE AND MUCUSLESS DIET

This cleansing program will purify the body so it may be healed. If you are overweight, this program will take you down to your normal body weight, and if you are underweight, it will bring you up to normal. The purpose of the entire program is to eliminate mucus from the body so that the patient is healed in a natural way.

After cleansing the body with this program, continue with the mucusless diet and other health-preserving procedures outlined in this booklet. In this way, you will not only help rid the body of disease-causing impurities but also maintain and build vibrant good health.

The Detoxification Procedure

The detoxification procedure we recommend is taken in part from Dr. N.W. Walker s book, *Fresh Vegetable & Fruit Juices*: To Detoxify

> Supreme cleanliness is the first step towards a healthy body. Any accumulation or retention of morbid matter or waste of any kind will retard our progress towards recovery. The natural eliminative channels are the lungs, the pores of the skin, the kidneys, and the bowels. Perspiration is the action of the sweat glands in throwing off toxins which would be injurious if retained in the body. The kidneys excrete the end products of food and body metabolism from the liver. The bowels eliminate not only the food waste but also waste matter known as body waste, in the form of used-up cells and tissues, the result of our physical and mental activities, which if not eliminated cause protein putrefaction resulting in toxemia or acidosis. The retention of such body waste has a much more insidious effect on our health than is generally suspected, and its elimination is one of the first steps toward perceptible progress toward health. The cleansing procedure will effect such elimination quickly, particularly for adults.

Juices

First thing in the morning we drink sixteen ounces of prune juice. The purpose of this prune juice is not primarily to empty the bowels, which, however, it will do anyway, but rather to draw into the intestines from every part of the body such toxic matter or body waste as may be there, and eliminate it through the bowels.

If nothing were done to replace in the body something in volume equal to the quantity of matter so eliminated, then the body would naturally be dehydrated to that extent. Therefore, we replace the toxic or acid material so removed by drinking fruit juices. This has an alkaline reaction on the system. There are various types of juice therapy apple, carrot, grape, citrus, tomato, etc. but use only the one chosen for the three days, and chew each mouthful thoroughly.

One of the most effective blood purifiers known is the common apple. Dr. Edward E. Shook states in Advanced Treatise in Herbology, Lesson number 30, page 307:

> There is no other remedial agent or herb in the whole range of known therapeutic agents, that can compare with the apple tree and, although it would be difficult to say which of its many virtues is the greatest, we suggest that its abundance of nascent oxygen compound is probably the main reason why it is such a precious food, blood purifier, and unfailing remedy for so many forms of diseases.

Other juices, of course, may be used, depending on the individual s preference and condition. Those who live in the citrus belt may use a combination, prepared fresh in the following proportions: four to six grapefruit, according to size; two to three lemons, according to size; and enough oranges to complete a total mixture of two quarts. The combination may be varied, as you may prefer. Grape juice may also be used; however, frozen grape juice is not recommended because many unacceptable additives are combined in nearly all cases.

The brands of juices sold in the health stores grown on unsprayed and organic soils, are definitely superior to other types that are sold in grocery stores; nevertheless, for many years we have seen many tremendous cures done with brands such as Church, Tea Garden,

Queen Isabella, and Welch. They still have great potency, but are not preferred when better juice is available.

After taking the sixteen ounces of prune juice first thing in the morning, within one half hour take an eight ounce glass (regular tumbler) of apple juice. Swish each mouthful thoroughly in the mouth (called chewing) so the saliva will mix with it, thereby getting all the nutritional and healing value from it. In fact, all meals should be eaten with little or no liquids so the food is chewed thoroughly enough to become a liquid by being mixed thoroughly with saliva, which is the key that opens the door to digestion.

We repeat, do not gulp the juice. In this way, there will be no danger of regurgitation to a weak stomach, but it will be very soothing and affable. By using the saliva properly, the healing program is greatly accelerated, for the rest of the digestive juices then are able to function properly instead of haphazardly. When desired, drink a glass of plain water (preferably a glass of distilled water), followed another half hour later with more apple juice. One gallon of apple juice is consumed throughout one day. This, of course, is an approximate and suggested dosage, as age, ability to hold liquids, etc., determine the capacity for each specific case. The alternating procedure, however, has proven to be the best way, with any juice you may choose for the therapy.

Do not eat anything all day, although if you become very hungry towards evening, you may take an apple or two with the apple juice, and carrots or celery with the carrot juice, or other suitable vegetables or fruits with the respective juice.

Other Aids

During the three-day cleanse, take one or two tablespoons of olive oil three times a day, to aid in lubricating bile and liver ducts, etc.

Breaking up the mucus during a juice cleanse generally causes constipation throughout these three days; use more prune juice, or take some of our Lower Bowel Formula, two or more capsules three times or more a day.

Begin the castor oil fomentation during this three-day juice cleanse.

Continue this detoxification for three consecutive days. Approximately three gallons of toxic lymph will have been eliminated from the body and will have been replaced by three gallons of juices. This will result in speeding up the re-alkalinizing of the system. If there is a jaundice condition or pain in the liver-gall bladder area, also use the Liver Gall-bladder Formula three times a day.

After the Three-Day Cleanse

Preparatory Fast: After the first three days of cleansing, if a person has the desire or ability to do so, it is always profitable to fast one to three days using only distilled water, then a day of juice, before returning to salads and other regular foods. Do not eat any heavy foods immediately after a cleansing period or after a fast, but add these to your diet gradually. This is the best and smoothest way to get back onto solid foods.

On subsequent days, begin taking vegetable juices and vegetables and fruit, preferably all raw. For breakfast, for example, eat fruit in season, sliced, chopped or grated, some honey for sweetening, and one or two tablespoonfuls of finely grated unsalted almonds sprinkled over. Also drink one or two glasses of fresh fruit or vegetable juices thirty minutes before or after eating fruit. For lunch, eat more fruit and one pint fresh raw vegetable juices. For dinner add any one of the salads given in the menus in *Mild Food Cook Book* (by Michael Tracy, Christopher Publications).

If there is the slightest tendency toward appendicitis, also take high enemas, two, three or more daily for one week or longer if necessary.

Cleansing Symptoms: As the cleansing begins the housecleaning process throughout the entire system, it will be accompanied by periodic aches and pains in the areas where the cleaning action is most acute and the wastage is loading the elimination system. There are times when you will feel very rough! Do not panic on your days after cleansing or during your periods of healing. In fact, the cleaning action may produce all the symptoms and effects of severe illness, but the patient should here act with knowledge and not blame the temporary problem condition onto the cleansing solution that is taking place for patience is required here, and much comfort should be derived in the realization that the healing process is well under way, and the sooner such discomforts come and are felt, the better.

This elimination and cleansing will not be accomplished instantaneously, and one should not expect these lifetime accumulations that are packed into the system to be miraculously squeezed and flushed out of the tissues and organs in some colonic fashion. This will all take time. You will have high days and low days, and these will take place in cycles. These cleansing sicknesses come in cycles of seven days, seven weeks, seven months, and seven years in most cases, and on each of these cyclic periods there will be healing and cleansing crises. As the toxic poisons break loose and are dumped into the blood stream so they can be eliminated from the physical body, you will feel pretty rough and quite frequently during a crisis you may feel worse than you ever did before starting the program but again, do not panic! These crises are, again, merely toxic poisons trying to get from your body (wherein they heavily load the excretory channels) and are doing you the favor of leaving as rapidly as possible (causing pain and discomfort in the elimination process). But the bad days will become fewer and fewer and the good days greater and greater, if you are faithful to the program. Professor Arnold Ehret s book *Mucusless Diet Healing System* (which can be purchased from most any health food store) may help you to understand some of the reactions you might experience while ridding the body of toxins, wastes, and mucus.

Do not be unduly alarmed if you feel somewhat weak during or after this detoxification. Nature uses our energies for a housecleaning within us, and we soon regain greater energy and vitality as a result of a cleaner and a healthier body. It is good to do the three-day cleanse monthly or several times a year.

The Mucusless Diet

We should not put mucus into the body faster than it can be eliminated. With this preventative diet, not only are the sinuses, the bronchi, and the lungs cleared, but also the constipating mucus (catarrh) in the tissues of the body from the head to the bottom of the feet.

Harmful or Mucus-Forming Foods

Secondary, denaturalized, or inorganic food substances are to be eliminated from the patient s diet.

Salt: For those who are accustomed to large amounts of salt, this may sound difficult, but if you will substitute coarsely ground pepper and savory herbs, adding powdered kelp, you will find that the craving for salt will immediately begin to disappear. The black pepper is a good nutritional herb and helps rebuild the body when used in its natural state. But, when pepper is cooked in food, the molecular structure changes, so it becomes an inorganic irritant (as high heat changes the cayenne, black pepper, and spices from organic to inorganic), and this is the only time when damage results. The use of salts of a vegetable or potassium base (such as Dr. Jensen s, Dr. Bronner s, and other various ones, which in some cases contain some sea salt) is all right, providing it is not overdone.

Eggs: No eggs should be eaten in any form.

Sugar and All Sugar Products: You may use honey, sorghum molasses, or blackstrap molasses, but no sugar of any type.

Meat: Eliminate all red meats from the diet. A little white fish once a week, or a bit of young chicken that has not been fed commercial food or inoculated with formaldehyde and other anti-spoilage serums, would be all right (as these are the higher forms of edible flesh), but do not use them too often.

Milk: Eliminate all dairy products, which includes butter, cheese, cottage cheese, milk, yogurt, etc. These are all mucus forming substances and, in most cases, are extremely high in cholesterol. As a substitute for butter or margarine (hardened vegetable oils, etc.), you can train your taste buds to enjoy a good, fresh, bland olive oil on vegetables, salads, and other foods and you will discover this is one of the choicest foods there is.

Flour and Flour Products: When flour is heated and baked at high temperatures, it changes to a mucus-forming substance. This is no longer a food, which means it has no life remaining therein. All wholesome food is organic, where unwholesome food or dead food is inorganic. This is the key to our whole mucusless program.

Supplements: Revitalizing and Healing Aids

Our supplement recommendations will build up strength in the body and start cutting the mucus out of the tissues and remove the catarrh from the system.

Cayenne: Take one teaspoonful of cayenne three times a day. Start gradually with 1/4 teaspoonful in a little cold water. Add 1/4 teaspoonful to this dosage every three days, until you are taking one teaspoonful three times a day (the graduated dosages will accustom your system to the pungency of the herb).

Honey and Apple Cider Vinegar: Place one tablespoonful of honey and one tablespoonful of vinegar in warm water, so that the honey will liquefy. Sip this amount three times a day so that at the end of the day a total quantity of three tablespoonfuls are consumed. This must be apple cider vinegar, do not use malts or other types of vinegars, as these are damaging to the body. The apple cider vinegar is medicinal and very beneficial.

Kelp: If there is any indication of a thyroid problem, you should use between ten and fifteen kelp tablets daily. Otherwise, two or more will keep the body in good condition as preventative nutrition. This can take the place of salt and helps build a new thyroid gland. Kelp powder can be used on salads and in other foods.

Molasses: Take one tablespoon three times a day of either sorghum or blackstrap molasses.

Wheat Germ Oil: Take one tablespoonful of a good, fresh wheat germ oil three times a day.

Dietary Suggestions: Regenerative Foods

If this diet is followed as outlined, we guarantee that after a short period of time you will have much more satisfaction from the foods we recommend for better health than you ever had from the food of your former diet. You will also come to your normal weight. If you are overweight, you will lose with this diet; and if you are underweight, you will gain after having passed your new low, as mucus must be expelled from the body before the good flesh can be restored.

Do not be concerned because this diet omits meat and the commercial types of protein, and don t worry about adding protein, as you will get all that you need in these foods. The gorilla is built on the same order as the human being, and he gets all the protein he needs from just fruit and nuts (and for the human, the greens will round out the body requirements). You can prove this program to yourself!

Morning

It is best not to break-the-fast (breakfast) until at least noon, except in cases of young or very active people. You will find that this will not be hard to do when you use items that we recommend (such as wheat germ oil, cayenne, etc.). These will lower the appetite while providing the need nutrition, so you will feel satisfied and will have taken these items even the second time during the morning because it is time to eat the regular noon meal but if (after taking the Lower Bowel Formula, wheat germ oil, cayenne, apple cider vinegar, honey, molasses, herbal teas, etc.), you have room left, are hungry, and want something to eat, the best food to start the day is a good low heated whole-grain cereal; however, this should be cereal in its wholesome state (with life in it). Or you may instead eat fresh fruits.

The cereal is prepared by first soaking the whole grain in water sixteen to twenty hours, then heating in stainless steel double boiler at a very low heat, 135 degrees or under, which can be done by pouring hot water over the grain and then applying low heat. It can also be prepared in a thermos bottle, as follows: Take a wide-mouth thermos bottle (pint, quart or whatever size you need for your size of family or individual); fill it in the early afternoon or evening one-third full of high-protein turkey red wheat; then finish filling the thermos bottle with boiling water (turning the container on its top and back once or twice, so that during the evening the water circulates completely into the bottom, or else some wheat in the bottom will not be treated).

When you uncover your vessel in the morning, after low heating the grain all night long, it should be ready for consumption. The wheat is popped open, is soft and very tasty (as none of the flavor has been lost in cooking); this procedure is still improved by presoaking. With a little oil or fresh butter added, it is a very delectable food. Some folks like to add cinnamon, nutmeg, allspice, etc.

Wheat contains all of the potential nutrient values needed in the human body. The wheat herb or wheat grass especially is a complete food, as it provides you with protein, calcium, and all the needed enzymes, vitamins, minerals, etc., to rebuild and regenerate the cell structure of your body. The grain is alive until it is killed in some chemical storage procedure, or high heat. The test for germane wheat (which is still in a wholesome state, having the life therein) is to plant is and see if it will grow.

This test is also valid for testing cooked wheat, and when low-heated in stainless steel, it will retain the life power and will grow! The foods, prepared in this manner, are organic; consequently, this is the manner that grains must be prepared for use. We are told in holy writ that all wholesome grains and herbs are for man, and grain is the staff of life, but it does not say that it is permissible to grind it to a face powder fineness or to heat it above 212 degrees F., and change the molecular structure from organic to inorganic, and thereby make it very mucus-forming. The results of man s inventions indicate otherwise. Sprout the grains if you wish, in preference to popping them open with moist heat.

Sprouted grains are excellent and nutritious but if you give a growing child a bowl of sprouts for breakfast, he is hungry in a short time, so a good serving of soaked, low-heated grain tastily prepared will stick to his ribs for hours. Alternate the wheat with barley, millet, buckwheat, rye, oat groats (whole, not rolled oats).

Noon

If you prefer only a light lunch, then have a tossed salad a salad as large as you want of mixed vegetables and leafy greens, using homemade olive oil dressing:

1 cup olive oil
2 tablespoonfuls apple cider vinegar
Pinch of herbs, black pepper, etc.

Make this dressing to your own taste, for there are so many varieties you can make avocado, onion, garlic, etc. but do not use the processed dressings of the commercial market.

Juices may be taken during the afternoon: carrot, grape, apple, etc. Dried fruits and nuts are very nourishing and beneficial, and the latter are better (as a whole protein) when used in combination with the garden greens. If a person has cancer or is inclined toward cancer, do not overdo eating protein, such as nuts. This is one thing that does damage to the pancreas and, in these cases, eat the nuts only in the morning. But stay away from peanuts and concentrate on almonds. A person with a cancerous condition should use from eight to ten almonds in the morning and the same at noon. But do not take any protein from evening time until the next morning, allowing sixteen to eighteen hours for the pancreas to clear and start to work on enzymes again. All protein should be taken early in the morning. And, of course, in cancer cases, never any secondhand or secondary protein, such as meats.

Proteins are a fad and are highly over-advertised. All fruits, vegetables, grains, nuts and seeds have protein in them. If you are eating a good live mucusless diet and wonder what to eat for protein, ask any gorilla. Their body organs are built just like a human s, and they live a number of years longer than humans. They are one of the strongest animals, for their weight, on the face of the earth. They are fruitarians, eating that which grows above the ground, fruits, grains, nuts and seeds. We enjoy underground roots and tubers, but they do not dig as we do; so with carrots, potatoes, beets, etc. added to the above-the-ground vegetation, we should do better than the gorilla.

We kill the cow to eat the steaks for the protein she gets from eating grass. Let s get our protein fresh and natural, not secondhand as from animal s flesh or from something in its dead state concocted by man. Commercial protein will work on the effect and give quick relief from certain ailments, but overuse of commercial types will overwork the pancreas and other glands, causing low blood sugar (hypoglycemia) and/or diabetes (high blood sugar). The natural live protein in foods on the mucusless program will be used as needed and the surplus discarded from the body naturally when not needed. The sedimentation of the commercial type of protein of lower vibration remains in the gland of the body and causes future trouble.

Regular meals can start off with a nice cup or bowl of potassium broth. Dehydrated vegetables in the form of potassium powder or broth can be purchased from most health stores or you can prepare your own. Some health books provide instructions for making potassium broth. You can add the leftover, savory vegetables and here you have one of the most exotic-tasting, low-heated vegetable soups that is imaginable. The broth starts the meal off, and is followed with salad. There are thousands of salad combinations, and with some investigation and experimentation, you will never run short of interesting ones.

After that, serve the low-heated vegetables (many types can be prepared with various savory herbs, and these can be removed from the low heat just before serving), and these will always be tasty and beneficial as long as they are low-heated and are still in a wholesome state. At least five to six vegetables should be eaten each day, of which two should be green, leafy ones. A small amount of bland oil (such as olive oil) added to the baked potato, baked squash, etc., is very good. If you are using cayenne regularly, you may use fresh butter on your vegetables. You can explore and concoct some very interesting, intriguing meals with a little daring and imagination, and you will never need to worry if you eat copiously until you are satisfied, and you will have all the nutrition that is needed for ample physical strength; use casseroles with whole grains.

You can prepare delicious casseroles with barley, rye, millet, wheat soaked as above and while low heating add fruits or vegetables, tasty herbs, etc. All lentils, beans, soys, etc., prepared this way are alive and good eating. Soys and most beans can be soaked for two or three days and then low-heated twelve to twenty hours adding onion, garlic, peppers, etc., during low-heating.

Do not drink liquids during mealtime. Mix food thoroughly with saliva. Wait one half hour after eating before drinking.

Evening

This is generally the heavy meal of the day, but you can reverse this at will if you like, eating the heavy meal maybe at noon, then the light meal with a salad at night. If you prefer a warm meal, start off with a cup of vegetable broth (regular potassium broth). The broth should be followed with a salad, then the main course is steamed vegetables that have been prepared at low-heat. Be sure to always cook in stainless steel, Pyrex, or some approved vessel, but never in aluminum!

Juice or nuts, dried fruits or fresh fruits are all excellent. Whenever you use a fresh fruit, use it alone, only one type of fruit at a time. When you want to eat some other type of fruit, wait for one half hour or more at least before eating it, and this will prove much easier on your digestive system. The mono-diet is also recommended for people on a healing routine. If the individual feels he is well and healthy, a fruit salad or mixed fruits at times is permissible.

APPENDIX C

FEVERS: THEIR CAUSES AND AIDS and THE COLD SHEET TREATMENT THERAPY

(Taken from *The Cold Sheet Treatment* by Dr. John R. Christopher)

When excess mucus, toxic materials, drug accumulations, poisons and other undesirable materials accumulate within the body, the body s natural reaction is to unload this material before it reaches a high enough level to cause death. The body then reacts with colds, small-pox, measles, chicken pox, or some other childhood disease. The first indication of disease that generally appears is a fever. An adult s first thought, when he sees that his child has a fever, is to hurry and lower the temperature to normal. This is a mistake because the fever is nature s way of letting us know the child has toxic material in his body which should be removed quickly. The fever should not be ignored, but we should work with it.

Fevers work in several ways. One is to raise enough temperature to move the bodybuilding materials from one part of the body to a malfunctioning area. A good example of this is when a baby is trying to cut teeth. The tooth bud appears, becomes swollen and red, painful and irritating; but there is not enough calcium in the mouth area to help get the tooth through. When there is no surplus calcium available, the fever goes higher and higher, and the infant often goes into convulsions. Time after time we have seen the fever drop quickly as organic calcium has been given to the child. The convulsion stops, and the child falls asleep (from fatigue). In a short time the tooth or teeth start popping through. If the parent uses medication to lower or suppress the fever and nothing else is done, he is merely working on the effect, and not going into the cause. In other words, he is stopping the attempt of a building process without assisting it to accomplish what the body is trying so hard to do.

A fever can be an aid and a blessing if worked with intelligently. But if it is fought against ignorantly, or ignored it is a killer . Our job in wholistic healing is to praise the fever and work with it, not fight against it. Fever is the thermostatic control of the body, letting us know a dangerous level of toxins has been reached. One should assist the fever to rebuild a malfunctioning area with the cleaning-feeding process. As the child develops a fever with a childhood disease, the body is doing two things; one is to draw healing aids from the body (if they are there), and the other is to discard or burn up unwanted materials. True, a fever must not be allowed to reach too high a level, so we will now show simple ways to help it to unload the unwanted toxic poisons, filth, and surplus mucus from the body.

When a child starts a fever, you are being given a signal that there is trouble in the child s system something needs attention. Trying to stop the fever without going to the cause is like bailing the water out of a sinking boat without plugging the hole in the bottom, which is, of course, the cause of its sinking. The water coming in is merely the effect.

The effect (or the fever) stems from the accumulation of toxins the child has received over a period of time, and these toxins must be neutralized and/or removed. The only thing we recommend as a natural way of gaining health are foods (herbs, which are foods) and helpful therapies that have been used for centuries. A pleasant herbal tea (red raspberry leaf and yarrow are specifics here) can be the answer when the fever is just starting, because it may be a minor condition or just a common cold. There may be a larger amount of toxic materials in some cases that require more help than just the herbal tea, and we will discuss this later on. For now, let s begin with a fever just showing itself.

The first thing we do is to check the bowels, and see if the child is constipated. If so, give the child some of the bowel formula as described in Appendix A, until bowels start to move freely. Many times a good bowel movement is all that is necessary to bring down a fever. Give a small child an herbal tea made of three parts china rhubarb (also called turkey or India rhubarb), two parts comfrey root, and one part licorice root one cup three times a day for children twelve years or older; one half cup for children eight to twelve years old. Vary this amount for younger children according to age.

We worry whether we should feed a fever and starve a cold or vice versa. Let s consider the actions of animals of the lower kingdom. They cannot read and don t understand old wives tales, so they are guided by God-given intuition, or have to depend on the inner feelings. When sick, they ignore food until they are well. If we force them to eat, we could easily kill them! During a fever, most people do not have an appetite, so do not force food on a sick child. Take all solid foods away and use only vegetable or fruit juice, preferably fresh (or unsweetened bottled) juice. Do not worry about your child falling over in starvation if he misses a meal or two. Too much food is generally the problem, causing fever and sickness simply an overloaded and constipated bowel area.

While the child is off solid foods, give him, in addition to juices, as many cups of red raspberry-leaf tea during the day as he can drink. Sweeten it with honey, and he will enjoy it, if the adult does not use the negative approach; i.e., Here is some more of that yucky herb drink. If the parent is wise, this can be a wonderful opportunity to get closer to the child and have a tea party, drinking the tea together. Both will benefit.

The red raspberry-leaf tea is high in a number of organic (natural and healing) minerals and vitamins and is a fine herbal liquid food for the body. This contains the wonderful nitrate of iron which has remarkable blood-making and regulating properties as well as astringent and contracting action on the internal tissues and membranes. It also contains pectin, malic and other organic acids, calcium, and potassium chloride, and sulphates. Here is a wonderful healing tea that is a great blessing.

This simple routine has aided many in cleaning up the body to a point that the fever drops back to normal before the day is over. Keep the child on juice and ripe fresh fruit for a day or two and then gradually onto the mucusless diet (see Appendix B). If the child is restless at night and does not sleep soundly, give the following warm herbal drink a short time before going to bed. Equal parts of catnip, peppermint and spearmint tea, sweetened with honey. Yarrow tea will break up a fever that is high and dry, by causing the child to sweat. Red raspberry leaf tea has been used and proven by many people, as explained above, but if not available, use yarrow or some other diaphoretic herb.

THE COLD SHEET TREATMENT

When your cold has advanced into a severe, chronic condition, or when you have no success with the first simple remedies, the Cold Sheet Treatment program is the next step you want to take. It successfully blends hydrotherapy with herbal therapy to clean out the body of its poisons and toxins. It works to break up systematic congestion, such as viral infections and pneumonias, that prevents normal bodily functions through the use of hot water and diaphoretic herbs. It is a very safe healing modality because it works with the body instead of against it.

Hydrotherapy has been used for centuries to heal the sick. It was once a common practice of doctors. The Romans built their famous baths in England not for pleasure bathing, but for health and treating illness. Hydrotherapy works well because the body is made up of over eighty percent liquid. Much of the fluids in the body are toxic, loaded with cholesterol, mucus, etc. When they are replaced in a natural way through hydrotherapy, with good liquid, we gain a healthy body.

An old story of the first Cold Sheet Treatment is as follows: Many years ago a peasant was heading home on foot, with miles to go. He was wracked with fever, colds, and lumbago. While crossing a stream, over a log for a bridge, he slipped and fell into the icy cold water and was drenched to the skin. It was a bitterly cold day, and the man had to walk home in the cold in his sloppy wet clothes. By the time he had arrived home, his clothes were nearly dried out. During his journey home the fever and heat of his body had raised to a point of a healing climax and reduced to a nearly normal temperature when he reached home. The lumbago and fever were gone, and he rejoiced. The next time he got lumbago and fever, he knew the cure he would return to the stream, dunk himself and walk home again. This story illustrates how hydrotherapy can help the body rid itself of toxins that slow down its bodily function, causing a person to become very weak and ill.

In the Cold Sheet Treatment program, your purpose is to build an artificial fever or increase the fever of your patient to a higher degree.

You are going to put your patient into a very hot bath to help build their fever. Using the heat of water and the heat of diaphoretic herbs, you will raise the temperature of your patient. This is done to bring an incubation condition into place or to cause the bacteria or viruses to multiple as rapidly as possible. These germs are God s gift to the sick because they speed up healing. They are like tiny scavengers, living off the toxins, mucus, poisons and filth of our bodies. To live they must eat, and the only thing they consume is the filth in our bodies. A germ cannot consume or live on a good, live cell structure. So when the body is clean from all toxins, disease germs leave because they have nothing more to live on. They are nature s perfect garbage men. We should work with them and not against them. With the moist incubation of a fever, the germs multiply faster and faster, devouring the mucus and waste cells of the body. When all the garbage is cleaned up out of our systems, they leave because they have nothing more to live on. But after cleansing the body of our sickness, or accumulated waste, the germ finishes its job and leaves us with a healing climax.

If we have taken inoculations or oral medications to kill germs, we have defeated the purpose of nature. It is like having a garbage man s strike in a large city. The city, unable to remove its waste because of the strike, is left with the accumulated stinking garbage on its streets, which not only congest traffic but make daily functions impossible. If you have ever been to a large city in these conditions, you know what an offensive filth this is to live in. Likewise, when we kill the bacteria or viruses in our bodies by medication, then we are left with all the rotting waste which congests our bodily functions. We still have our original congestion plus the corpses of all the germs we have just killed with our inoculation.

This causes our heart to labor harder to pump the sludge through our system, pulling calcium from wherever it can to help this extra labor. This causes a calcium deficiency, which can cause rheumatic fever (causing a rheumatic heart and a weakened body) that can even develop into polio, stroke, multiple sclerosis, muscular dystrophy, etc. The rheumatic fever leaves a calcium weakness that can lie dormant for years until an additional loss of calcium will trigger one of these maladies to develop.

Instead of using antibiotics or aspirins to reduce your patient s temperature, you should build a fever as fast as possible with moisture. You can run the temperature as high as you want without any harm if you follow one important principle. The key for keeping your patient s fever from doing harm is moisture. As you build a fever in your patient, you must make sure your patient is drinking fluid, a diaphoretic tea, every ten to fifteen minutes. This will keep their fever moist, and your patient will not have dry heat which can cause febrile damage to the body, such as infantile paralysis, brain fever, etc. As long as you administer fluids to your patient, you will not have to worry about the damage that a dry heat fever can cause. Moist heat is life; it is the Garden of Eden. Dry heat is death; it is the desert. And the more your patient sweats, the better because the perspiration will bring toxic poisons and waste out of the body. Always remember, fevers are necessity to helping the body rid itself of disease. Doctors now recognize that the body will build a fever to counteract the viruses it encounters.

To do this program properly, you should have at least two people. This treatment takes time, and is best to do in the evening so your patient can sleep through the night after the treatment. It is wise to make all your preparations before you proceed with the Cold Sheet Treatment, then your full attention can be devoted to your patient during the therapy. Before beginning, read through each step carefully, then prepare the preparations needed. This will allow you to proceed for one step to the next step easily and concentrate on the needs of your patient.

Items you will need:

Garlic (fresh)	10—15 cloves or more
Diaphoretic herb	8 ounces or 225 grams
Cayenne Pepper	1 ounce or 28.35 grams
Dry mustard powder	1 ounce or 28.35 grams
Ginger powder	1 ounce or 28.35 grams
Apple cider vinegar	16 ounces or 1/2 liter
Distilled water	1 gallon or 4 liters
Fruit juice	1 gallon or 4 liters

Olive oil 1 ounce or 30 ml.
Petroleum jelly 4 ounces or 113. 4 grams
Gauze or cotton strips
2 large cotton socks
Natural sponge
Enema bucket or bag
Rectal syringe
Towels
Bucket or ice chest
Safety pins
Plastic or rubber sheet for bed
Cotton sheet bedding
Several natural fiber blankets (wool, cotton, linen or silk)
1 Double cotton sheet
Cayenne extract (in case of shock)
Pots or Pans (stainless steel, glass or corning ware)
Strainer (stainless steel)
Measuring cup
Cold Sheet Treatment Procedure

Step One: Cleansing Enema

To start the Cold Sheet Treatment, you will want to help the body cleanse out any toxicity that may be preventing it from regaining its health. To do this, you will need to give your patient an enema using catnip, sage, red raspberry, or some similar herb, but preferably catnip. You will want to administer this enema cold. A cold enema will cause the anus and rectal area to contract and retain the fluid until it warms to body temperature. It will then cause the area to relax and void the fluid and fecal matter. If the patient has a fever, the body will hold the enema longer until the fluid reaches the body s heated temperature. This allows the liquid to stay in the body longer, permeating more dried waste matter and loosening it.

Do not use enemas except in the case of emergencies. When used regularly they can become habit forming; the body can become dependent on enemas for its bowel movements. The use of enemas in this program is only as an emergency. You want to get the bowel to work on its own.

Step Two: Garlic Injection

In herbology an injection is never with a needle; it is a syringe type application into an already existing orifice of the body, i.e. the rectum, ears or nose. Insert the prepared garlic injection into the rectum with a syringe. Use the full pint for an adult and less for a child. Have your patient retain the injection as long as possible before voiding. Keep your patient well covered while he or she is retaining the injection. You will find it is easier to retain the liquid if the patient is lying on a slant board or has their buttocks elevated with pillows.

Step Three: Hydrotherapy

After your patient has voided the garlic injection, help him or her into the hot bath prepared with the diaphoretic herbs. Have the water as hot as your patient can possibly tolerate. Cayenne, dry mustard and ginger will increase the perspiring of the patient by opening the pores wide, allowing heat and moisture to be brought in, and this is very important. You will want to build the fever as fast as possible with moisture. Dry fever is a killer, causing infantile paralysis, brain fever, etc., but moist fevers can go much higher. Used properly, moist fevers work with the disease germs in removing the sickness from the body. They can only do good as the Maker of the human body intended.

Step Four: Diaphoretic Tea

To assist increasing the fever, you should give your patient a diaphoretic tea. Because your patient is in a hot tub of water, they will become very thirsty. Do not give them cold drinks. Cold drinks will inhibit the body s ability to perspire and produce a disease-fighting fever. Instead, give them cups of a hot diaphoretic tea, such as yarrow or another type. You will want to stay with only one type of tea. Have your patient drink as much as possible. This will keep the patient from a dry fever. It will also increase the body s circulation which will help remove the toxicity from the body, and it will open the body s pores which will eliminate the toxicity. You should give them a cup to drink about every ten to fifteen minutes.

During this sweating scene, your patient may get light-headed and feel like fainting. If so, place a cold towel or washcloth on the forehead. You should leave the patient in the hot bath as long as possible, at least forty-five minutes (may reduce for a small infant). You will know when to get a child out by when perspiration starts to bead up on the face. When perspiration starts to show on the head of the child, then you know that the heat has circulated throughout the body and has done a good job. At this point, you can give them ten or fifteen more minutes. The duration of the bath will depend on the sickness, the patient s tolerance, and his or her age. If the sickness is severe, you will want a longer duration. When your patient is ready to leave the tub, you will need to lift him or her out, as they will be unable to support themselves. Fainting can occur when you pull your patient out of the bath. Keep a cayenne tincture on hand in case your patient goes into shock.

Step Five: Cold Sheet Therapy

After you have helped the patient out of the bath, wrap the large double cotton sheet, dripping wet from being soaked in ice cold water, around the standing patient. This cold sheet will feel extremely refreshing to your sweating patient. With just the head and feet protruding, pin the sheet down at the side. Help your patient into the prepared bed that has been covered with plastic and with a cotton sheet. Then place dry cotton sheet covers over the patient while they are still wrapped in the cold sheet. Add additional natural fiber blankets over the top of the sheet for warmth and to continue the sweating routine.

You will want natural fibers rather than synthetic materials because synthetic cloth does not breathe. Synthetic materials will not allow oxygen, the breath of life, to get into the body. Approximately sixty percent of all breathing done by the human body is done from the neck down through the skin, and if the skin is covered with synthetic material, which will not permit breathing, your patient will eventually suffocate.

Step Six: Garlic Paste

With your patient lying down in bed, thoroughly massage their feet from the ankles down with olive oil. Allow as much of this oil to be absorbed into the skin as possible, covering the sole, sides and entire foot area. Make the garlic paste by mashing the garlic (or pressing it) into a small bowl, then add the petroleum jelly. The low vibration petroleum jelly will not be absorbed into the skin, as will anhydrous lanolin or a vitamin ointment. The petroleum jelly holds the garlic in suspension whereas the high vibration ointments would be absorbed and leave the garlic exposed to the bare skin which will blister it. After you have massaged each foot, prepare a strip of cotton that is wide enough to cover the bottom of the foot with 1/2 inch of the garlic paste. When this is done, place the strip of cotton with the paste on the sole of the foot, then take a roll of two inch gauze and gently wrap the foot to secure the strip of garlic to the foot. With this in place, gently pull over the foot and gauze bandage a large white cotton or wool sock to hold everything in place.

Do not allow the paste to get up on the sides or on top of the foot. Put it only on the sole. This is where the major reflex area (zonal therapy) is located on the bottom of the foot. In this area all the nerves from the whole body end, allowing one to stimulate organs and other areas of the body through the feet. When the garlic paste is applied to the sole of the feet, it will disperse its oxygen-carrying power (the breath of life) throughout the body via the zonal nerves for healing.

Put the bandaged feet back under the cold, wet sheet and pin the bottom of the sheet together so that the patient will be in a wet sack. You will want to use a large double sheet instead of small because it will allow your patient to roll or turn around without being too closely confined.

Step Seven: Sound Sleep

In most cases, your patient will sleep soundly all night in the cold sheet. You do not have to worry about them wanting to get up to urinate because of the large quantity of tea they drank. While the body is in the cold, wet sheet, the subconscious mind will build an artificial fever to warm the body. From this incubation process, the patient s body will use the fluid from the ingested teas and accumulated moisture from their bath to warm the outside of their wet body. This process causes perspiration and draws heavily on the body for moisture to produce its heat, leaving no desire to urinate. While this is being done, the body breaks loose old toxins, drugs and medicines, mucus, and poisons which have accumulated and carries them out of body through the sweating process. Your patient will lie all night in a deep sleep, sweating out the poisons of their body.

As the toxins are voided from the body, your patient s rest will be better than ever before due to the cleansing of the body. When your patient wakes in the morning, they will be refreshed and invigorated from having such a thorough cleanse. The large, white sheet, which was wrapped around your patient, will no longer be wet. Your patient s fevered body has dried it out during the night. In addition, it should no longer be white. It will often be stained with toxic residue secreted out of the body during the night. This program has pulled out of the system the dead, inorganic minerals which have been stored by the body. These deposits of poisons have been causing side effects for the patient for years. Now they will be stains on the sheet or dye from old drugs and toxins from as far back as childhood. The dye from these poisons will be various shades and colors from pastel to dark.

It is far better to have these inorganic drugs and poisons on the sheet rather than slowing down the activities of the body. This program has been used successfully in removing the cravings for nicotine, alcohol, as well as other drug addictions. However, the patient must want to have this aid and must cooperate with the program.

Step Eight: Sponge Bath

After your patient wakes from their deep sleep, take them out of the bed and sponge them down thoroughly with a warm mixture of one part apple cider vinegar and one part distilled water. You will probably want one quart of solution, so use approximately one pint of each. This removes any remaining toxic residue from the outer layers of the skin. It is very important that you do not leave the toxic residue on the skin. Sponging off the body will allow the skin to breathe. If the pores remain plugged with residue, it is as if the doors and windows of a building are closed and stagnation sets in.

Your patient will now feel as though all the weight of the world has been lifted off their shoulders with the poisons and toxins removed. They will be anxious to start their new life with ambition and turn the world into a better place because they feel better. Put fresh clothing on them and put fresh bedding on your patient s bed. Now, you will want to have your patient go back to bed and relax for awhile to regain their strength. This treatment taxes the body s energy so your patient will need to take it easy for a day or two. All the glands are used in this treatment, and it will take time for the body to restore its energy reserve.

Step Nine: Juice Therapy

Your patient should by this time have a desire for something to drink or to eat. This is a critical moment for your patient; what they eat will either retain or cause them to loose their health. They may even have cravings from the past. They may desire a steak, a full meal, processed beverages, ice cream, creamy pastries, or other junk food. Do not respond to these desires. Instead, give your patient fresh fruit or vegetable juices (juices from Dr. N.W. *Walker s Fresh Vegetable and Fruit Juices* or wheat grass drink in *School of Natural Healing*) or bottled or fresh grape juice, apple juice, etc, with no additives. Each mouthful of juice should be swished or chewed thoroughly to mix it with the saliva for good assimilation. In addition, chewing your juice will prevent an unpleasant sugar reaction if your patient is hypoglycemic or diabetic.

Do not mix the your patient s juices, but let them drink (chew) as much of one kind that they desire or feel comfortable with. If a change of juice is desired, wait at least one half hour before using a different one. After a few hours, if your patient is really hungry, let them have a little ripe fresh fruit, but it must be chewed to a liquid before swallowing. During the day it is good for your patient to have as much distilled water as desired and some good herb teas. You can add a little honey to the teas if your patient desires it. It is really best when possible to keep the patient on juice therapy for one to three days to allow thorough cleansing of the digestive organs before going into the mucusless diet.

Step Ten: Teaching Your Patient

After a bad siege of body malfunction, it is wise to instruct the patient why they were in this condition, and what to do from this point on to prevent a reoccurrence of the disease. Your patient may get immediate relief from the Cold Sheet Treatment program, but if they do not change their health habits, they will not be able to retain their health. To work on just the effect and give relief is not a complete program. This sickness has been given as an education to teach your patient how to clean up a bad condition as well as how to keep the body in such a condition that there will be no reoccurrences. This is knowledge turned into power the power for a better life, a higher vibrating body , a body that is clean (God will not dwell in an unclean tabernacle), and an instrument so well-tuned that it can experience the joy of living and can even tune into The Great Universal Mind. The power of clairvoyance and intuition, can come to such a clean body. After teaching your patient the way to receive health and hold it, they may often return gratitude and thanks by becoming the student to learn more of the healing program, and thus become a helper, teacher and instructor to assist others in learning and understanding the natural way of life.

Cold Sheet Treatment Preparations

Iced Sheet

Take a large double sheet and soak in ice water. You can use a large bucket or ice chest filled with ice and water. Saturate the sheet in the water and place the bucket or chest next to tub.

Diaphoretic Tea

Prepare a gallon of diaphoretic tea. This can be any good sweating herb, preferably yarrow. But it can also be blessed thistle, camomile, pleurisy root, boneset, thyme, hyssop, garden sage, catnip, spearmint, or any other good diaphoretic herb.

For one gallon:

1 cup, (8 ounces or 225 grams)	Diaphoretic herb
1 gallon or 4 liters	Distilled water

Preparation: Pour boiling water over herbs, cover and allow to steep (not boil) in a warm place 30 minutes. Strain and sweeten with honey if desired. Keep warm until used.

Garlic Paste

To prepare a garlic paste for an adult, use 1 part garlic and 1 part petroleum jelly. Reduce the amount of garlic for a child or small infant to 1 part garlic to 3 parts petroleum jelly. For an adult, you will want about 1 cup of paste.

For an adult:

one half cup or 115 grams	Garlic, crushed
one half cup or 115 grams	Petroleum jelly

For a small child:

one eighth cup or 28.5 grams	Crushed garlic
one half cup or 115 grams	Petroleum jelly

Preparation: Crush or finely grate peeled garlic cloves. Blend with an equal amount of petroleum jelly.

Hot Bath

Fill a bathtub full of hot water, as hot as possible (without blistering or scalding your skin). The following is a water temperature guide.

Possible injury	above 50° C	above 122° F
Painfully hot	42.8 to 46° C	110 to 120° F
Very hot	40 to 42.8° C	104 to 110° F
Hot	38 to 40° C	100 to 104° F
Warm	35 to 38° C	92 to 100° F
Tepid	27 to 34° C	80 to 92° F
Cool	21 to 27° C	70 to 80° F
Cold	13 to 21° C	55 to 70° F
Very Cold	0 to 13° C	32 to 55° F

Burn Potential

Water Temperature	Exposure Time
158° F. (70° C.)	1 second
149° F. (65° C.)	2 seconds
140° F. (60° C.)	3 to 5 seconds
135° F. (57° C.)	10 seconds
133° F. (56° C.)	15 seconds
127° F. (53° C.)	60 seconds
124° F. (51° C.)	3 minutes

Add to the water, according your tolerance, one or all of the following diaphoretic herbs, ginger being the most mild, then dry mustard, with cayenne as the most stimulant.

1 ounce or 28.35 grams	Cayenne
1 ounce or 28.5 grams	Ginger powder
1 ounce or 28.5 grams	Dry mustard powder or seed (ground)

Bed with Plastic

Prepare a bed by placing a rubber or plastic sheet over the mattress, with a cotton sheet over it. Have several natural blankets on hand, such as wool or cotton.

Enema

4 tbl.	Catnip, Sage or Red Raspberry cut or powdered herb
1 qt.	Distilled Water

Preparation: Bring distilled water to a boil and pour over cut herb. Steep for 30 minutes. Strain the herb and set in refrigerator until tea is cool. Pour tea into enema bucket or bag. Lubricate the end of the enema hose to be inserted into the rectum. For child, use half the amount.

Garlic Injection

1 cup or 1/4 liter	Apple cider vinegar
1 cup or 1/4 liter	Distilled water

3 or more cloves Garlic

Preparation: Combine vinegar and water. Grate, squeeze through garlic press, or puree in a blender 3 cloves of garlic until finely crushed. Blend in water and vinegar mixture. Put mixture into syringe and check flow. If flow is very loose, add additional crushed garlic. Continue adding as much garlic as you can, making sure the mixture flows from syringe without clogging. The more garlic you can use without clogging the syringe, the better injection you will have.

APPENDIX D

THE INCURABLES PROGRAM

(Taken from the booklet *Curing the Incurables* by Dr. John R. Christopher)

There are no incurable diseases, but at times there are incurable patients. The Creator has given herbs and assisting wholistic therapies for every type of body malfunction. If they are used, benefits will come. But if they are not used as directed, they can be of no aid.

Over the years, we have put together a healing program that has done miracles for those who have conscientiously used it. It has even brought people who were supposedly on their death beds back to a full and active life. Yet, this program yields no results unless the instructions are followed carefully.

No one can truly tell a patient that he or she has just so many days, weeks, or months to live. The scriptures plainly say that everything moves in its time and season; there is an hour to be born and an hour to die. We have seen cases where the person was told that he had only a few days to live, and many of these people are alive and well today, because they had faith to turn to the natural ways of healing and have been healed.

For example, the parents of a small child, about eighteen or twenty months old, were told by their family practitioner that the child would not live until morning. He had a severe case of pneumonia. They lived in a rural area too far from a hospital. It was sub-zero weather, and the doctor said the child would die en route to the hospital by car. He explained that he would return the next morning and sign the death certificate. The parents had the hope and faith that the child could be saved. After the doctor left, and after much telephoning, they were referred to us at about midnight. When we arrived and gave him natural healing aids, the child was soon sleeping comfortably. The next morning when their doctor came to sign the death certificate, the child was sitting up having some juice for breakfast.

We have seen cases where the patients were lying helpless on their bed so sickly they could not feed themselves and were waiting for death at any moment. These people, by correctly utilizing this wholistic healing program, are alive, active and well today.

Even when a person is near death and suffering great pain, the natural healing procedure can be used to reduce the pain and give comfort in the last hours. Every one of God s children deserves help to ease unbearable conditions with helpful but harmless natural aids.

This program has been used for many different malfunctions with great success in nearly every case: multiple sclerosis, muscular dystrophy, stroke, deteriorating bones, curvature of the spine, locked arthritis joints, tumors and cysts in nearly all parts of the body. We have seen great improvement reduction in pain and often complete healing in these cases which are supposedly incurable. As in all natural healing, this program works with the body to cure itself and does not use any addicting medications or harmful therapies to affect health.

DR. CHRISTOPHER S INCURABLES PROGRAM

The patient may have suffered in their chronic condition for a long period of time. Because of the years of improper eating, the body is now suffering from malnutrition. This is because food is not being assimilated, causing starvation of the body s cells. It is not the amount of food that has been eaten matters, but the quality and how well it has been assimilated. We may take a healthy quantity of food into our bodies, but only that which has been properly assimilated can be utilized for rebuilding and repairing cells and malfunctioning areas. Proper assimilation is acquired by drinking the solid foods and chewing the liquid food. This is an old and true axiom. What this means is we should thoroughly chew our solid foods which mixes the saliva with the food until it becomes liquid, and then we drink it. The liquid foods must be swished (or chewed) in the mouth, then swallowed. The saliva thoroughly mixed with the foods is the key that opens up the doors of digestion. Without mixing saliva with the food, the balance of the digestive juices are not activated for good assimilation. By gulping or inhaling our food without properly mixing saliva with it, we get only eight to ten percent of its value. By properly chewing, we can raise this to forty or forty-five percent. The remainder is generally cellulose or indigestible fiber. We not only receive better health but also save money.

Food is one of our largest expenditures. If we can get four to six times better assimilation and use four to six times less food, we are saving a lot of money! By this simple method alone, which gives better assimilation, we gain superior health and a happier life. With one fourth or one third of the food we have been used to eating, we can receive much more power and energy. Remember, a large part of attaining good health results from chewing both solid foods and liquid foods.

The First Week of Wholistic Aid

Food: Many people feel that without three large meals of solid food each day they will starve, shrivel up and blow away! Dr. N.W. Walker in his book, *Fresh Vegetable and Fruit Juices*, and Johanna Brandt in her book, *The Grape Cure*, both show that juices alone sustain health for a long time in addition to healing the body.

The following suggestions are for a persisting chronic condition, not an acute one requiring emergency treatments. For the first week, drink as much fresh carrot juice as desired. Some people are satisfied with a quart while others need a gallon or more. Drink by chewing an eight-ounce glass or more each hour during the day for six days the first week.

Drink one cup or more of slippery elm gruel each day. The liquid can be as thin or thick as desired. With this herb, you take the powder and carefully mix it with enough water (preferably distilled) to form a paste because it does not mix easily. Then thin it to desired consistency by adding more water. A little honey can be added if preferred. In addition, drink one cup or more of comfrey leaf or root tea each day. Twenty minutes before or after drinking the juice, tea or gruel, drink as much steam-distilled water as desired.

Herbal Formulas: During the first week, we also help the body rebuild by the use of herbal formulas. One cup or more of the Complete Tissue Formula which should be used for the rebuilding of cells in flesh, cartilage and bones. Also, take one cup three times a day of Blood Stream Formula, to help the body build healthy, disease free blood.

Take the following every day with some liquid:

- Two or more capsules of the Lower Bowel Formula, three times a day. This is for regularity, as solid foods are not cleansing the bowels.
- Two or more capsules of the Nerve Formula, three times a day. This formula contains herbal nervines.
- Two or more capsules of the Pancreas Formula, three times a day. This assists the Lower Bowel Formula.
- Two or more capsules of the Herbal Calcium Formula, three times a day. This formula is a good source of organic, assimilable calcium.

Breathing With Depth: The Lord put into us the breath of life, but we have to keep it there. Shallow breathing is not much life, but full breathing is the full breath of life. Learn to breathe deeply, as is taught in yoga, to get the breath of life into the upper lobes of the lungs.

Clothing: Synthetic cloth strangles and chokes the body and is a barrier to oxygen the breath of life. We should use only natural fibers for the clothes we wear and also for our bed covers. Never use synthetic cloth for straining herbal drinks or for fomentations and bandaging. Use only natural fibers such as cotton, wool, linen or silk.

Releasing Static Electricity: Walk or jog barefooted on the lawn to get rid of the static electricity in the body and to allow new electrical vibration to come from the atmosphere. This is pure universal electricity that operates all the parts and organs of the body. It cannot come if static electricity is present, which should be grounded through the feet to keep a continual flow on hand.

Three Oil Massage: For the first two days, massage the patient with castor oil, using a clockwise circular motion from the top of the head to the bottom of the feet, always working toward the heart. The next two days use olive oil, and the last two days of the week massage with wheat germ oil.

By using the skin as a filtering agent, the castor oil cleans and flushes the skin. It also goes into the blood stream, aiding in the removal of mucous and toxins from the inner body. The olive oil is a complete food itself and will penetrate into the body to feed and rebuild muscles, flesh and the entire system. Wheat germ oil is a healing oil, high in vitamin E, valuable in rejuvenating the body.

On the seventh day, rest the patient, using no foods, herbs or juice, only steam-distilled water as much as is desired.

Sunbath: Immediately after the massage, have the patient take a sunbath each day in the nude, not through glass but in direct sun. Only allow two minutes on the front and two minutes on the back the first day. Add two minutes front and back each day but no more. In six days you will be up to twelve minutes front and twelve minutes back. Do not sunbathe between eleven in the morning and one o clock in the afternoon, that is, not at high noon. If it is a cloudy or cold day, use a sunlamp, but do not allow a burn.

The sun is the world s greatest doctor but must be used by building up the exposed time in the sun gradually so as to not burn. Do not be alarmed by articles in national publications each spring, warning people to avoid sunbathing, saying it is cancer-forming. The sun cannot cause cancer. When you do not gradually increase the use of it but lie in the sun for long lengths of time and burn, certainly it is dangerous for it will cause a severe toxic burn. But it is not cancer-forming. If cancer is already in the bloodstream and the body, the sun can ripen it and bring it to the surface, but that is the only way skin cancer can result from the sun.

Ask any Aborigine, Native American or member from any tribal area where only a loin cloth, if anything, is worn. Although their bare skin is exposed constantly to the sun year around, they have no cancer. If any of them develop skin cancer, it is because they have been eating a diet of modern processed food for a sufficient period of time to get the body into a toxic condition.

John N. Ott s book, *Health and Light*, explains the benefits of healing with light. This research scientist explains how natural sunlight is a food or nutrient and can cure many ills and keep us well, while the wrong kind (artificial light) can make us ill. Ott shows how certain ailments respond to a daily treatment of full spectrum light.

Baths: Each day the patient should have a hot bath followed by a cold shower or cold bath. No soap should be used for the bath unless it is a good biodegradable body cleanser. Each day before the bath, give a dry skin brushing (always toward the heart), using a natural bristle brush (not nylon). Sixty percent of all of our breathing is done through the skin, so it must be kept clean with water and brushing. The skin is our second set of kidneys and must be kept in good condition.

Herbal Fomentations: We use an herbal fomentation each night of the six days of the week. It should cover the head area (hair line), down the spine, all the way down to the end of the tailbone. Make a cap fit down to the ears (or use a cotton or wool skull cap) and stitch a flannel strip four or five inches wide down the back over the spine area. After wetting the fomentation cloth with Complete Tissue Formula tea and lightly wringing it out, cover it with a plastic over the head (shower cap, etc.) and a strip down over the spine. The moisture will go into the body and not the bedding or mattress. The fomentation down the back can be held into place with sweat shirt and shorts.

To aid the motor nerve and spinal cord, use our Nerve Formula, inserting with an eye dropper four to six drops of oil of garlic and four to six drops of this herb tincture into each ear six nights a week. Plug the ears with cotton overnight, and on the seventh day flush out the ears with half and half warm apple cider vinegar and distilled water. Repeat this each week during the program.

Zonal Foot Massage (Reflexology): If possible, use zonal therapy on the feet three times a week, leaving one day in between such as Monday, Wednesday, Friday, or Tuesday, Thursday, Saturday. Zonal therapy will greatly speed up the program. You may find a number of good books on zone therapy at libraries or health food stores.

The Second Week

The second week will be the same as the first except, instead of fresh carrot juice, substitute apple juice. Freshly made apple juice is best. If you do not have a juicer or fresh apples are not available, use a bottled apple juice that has had nothing added. Use canned only in an emergency. Do not use frozen juice, as nearly all frozen juices have additives. During this second week use the three-oil massages, sunbaths, zonal therapy, fomentations, etc. With the sunbaths add two minutes front and back onto the final total of the last week.

On the day of fast, there may be some physical reactions because you have reached a cleansing cycle. Toxic poisons break up in the body, accumulating for disposal and causing some upset. Do not be alarmed, for with some people it is more pronounced than with others. This same cyclical reaction can happen in any healing program in the third week, seventh week, seventh month and seventh year. The longer spasms occur in the major cycles and can be more pronounced, by far, than the minor cycles. If a cleansing crisis occurs during this short time, be happy with it and smile through the tears, for it shows the program is working well.

The Third Week

Again repeat the full complete program, except instead of carrot or apple juice, during the third week use grape juice. Freshly made is best from dark grapes (concord preferred), juice from organically grown grapes found in some health stores, or any of the standard brands in bottles such as Welch s, Church s, etc. Be sure in the bottled juice there are no additives (preservatives or sugar). It can be pasteurized but not frozen.

The Fourth Week and On

Continue to rotate the three juices each week as before. This program is life- sustaining as the patient is taking rapid-healing and wholesome food. If the patient desires more solid food, just add one solid meal each day. This meal should consist of a good fresh vegetable combination salad (as many raw fresh vegetables as you desire). If a salad dressing is desired, use a natural one, such as one made with fresh olive oil, apple cider vinegar or lemon juice, and, if desired, a small amount of honey, grated fresh onion and garlic to taste, savory salad herbs, coarse freshly ground black pepper, etc.

A small serving of presoaked, low-heated grain may also be added. This is done by taking the whole uncracked grain (wheat, rye, millet, buckwheat, barley or whole oat groats) and soaking it with distilled water. Soak in a cool place so it won t sour, up to twenty hours depending on the hardness of the grain. Then low-heat it in a stainless steel or Pyrex double boiler for twelve to fourteen hours. Use a food thermometer and do not allow the temperature to rise over 130 degrees F. If you use a crockpot, equip it with a dimmer switch or some other type of control so it will not overheat.

In whole live grain you have nearly every known vitamin and mineral known to mankind, but this live food must not be killed by overheating. Professor Arnold Eheret and the Rodale Press have both advised against the use of grain because of its acidity. In its hard state, grain is generally a pH 5. By using presoaked, low-heated grain we raise it from the objectionable pH 5 to a 7 pH which is easily assimilated.

The salad and grains must be chewed thoroughly until they become liquid before swallowing. These additions can be used in the healing routine as long as is desired. On this type of food a person can live to a ripe, healthy old age. As the individual improves in health, a larger variety of fruits, vegetables, grains, nuts and seeds can be used. Later, all the lentils, beans and harder seed types with longer soaking and more low-heating can be added. With these, and low-heated grains, delicious casseroles may be created. Also, potatoes which are steamed or slow baked using their skin are a very good food. Use fresh olive oil on them and coarse ground black pepper and, if desired, chives and/or other herbal seasoning.

Use no salt, sugar, eggs, meats, bread, milk or milk products. In a short time you will find the hidden hunger will leave by using the food recommended. The cravings will disappear and will be replaced with a cozy, unbloated, satisfied fullness that will bring ease and peace.

CASE HISTORIES

A young man came to us with advanced curvature of the spine. He had been told that the case was so bad his back would have to be broken in several places to fuse it but with no guarantee as to results. He tried our program, and in shortly over six months, he had a back that was straight and perfect. He had regained the three inches he had lost with the curvature and is now 6 6" as before his curvature. He could now go back to yoga and the sports, which he enjoyed.

In Mesa, Arizona, a young man in his middle twenties was brought into our lecture hall in a wheel chair. He was badly crippled with a combination of polio and arthritis. He was lifted out of his chair and placed on a pile of pillows. Looking at him, you could see the severe pain he was suffering.

During the lecture we discussed the program we have just outlined. After the lecture, he said he would like to try it. A practical nurse from another town offered to take him to her home and help him get well.

They followed the routine accurately and one year later we saw him again. Just before the lecture started, in the same hall as the year before, this young man walked down the aisle to the front of the hall and asked to speak. We granted him the permission. In his short talk he advised the people to listen to the lectures and put them to use. He described how just one year before he had listened to this lecture in the hall as he sat on pillows. He had gained the desire to start on this natural program. Prior to that night he had been told he would never be out of the wheelchair unless it was to be in a hospital bed the rest of his days.

With the help of the kind nurse, he was now able to walk so well that he was traveling on foot, house to house selling, to pay off his large hospital and doctor bills. As he walked back to his seat, he had tears of gratitude in his eyes.

There are many outstanding cases but these two can give you a picture of what can be done with the good, wholistic program. Use it carefully and accurately for complete, long-lasting health.

APPENDIX E

SKIN ERUPTIONS AND OTHER SKIN DISEASES

When rashes and pus eruptions of disease break out on the body, do not stop them. This is poison in the body that should be released. Keeping the skin from breaking out is defeating nature s efforts for a complete healing and housecleaning. The larger the break-out of rashes (chicken pox, measles, etc.) the better off the child! If the body is in a fairly clean condition and you follow these suggestions of natural therapy you may see that the rash is not as heavy as you might expect because there was not a great amount of toxic waste to eliminate. In other cases the body can be well covered with the dermal or dermatitis break-out. There is nothing to fear as long as you are willing to work with nature. To speed up the cleaning of the body, we work with the fever by assisting it to do its job. A moist fever is a healing fever, and a dry one can be a killing or crippling one.

The idea is to build an artificial fever (or increase the fever they already have) to a higher degree. This is being done to bring an incubation condition into place, to cause the disease germs to multiply as rapidly as possible. The germs are God s gift to the sick to be used to speed up a healing. The germ is a scavenger that lives on toxins, mucous, poisons and filth. They are nature s perfect garbage men. We should work with them, not against them. With the moist incubation they multiply faster and faster. To live they must eat and the only thing they can consume is the filth of the body. When all the garbage is cleaned up they leave, because they have nothing more to live on.

A germ cannot consume or live in good live cell structure. If they could then we should have a great fear! But after cleaning out the body of our sickness, which is accumulated waste, the germ finishes its job and leaves us with a healing climax.

If we take shots, inoculation and/or oral medication to kill the germs, we have defeated the purpose of nature. It is like having a garbage man s strike in a large city. We have seen this several times in our travels, and in one large city it was estimated that three thousand tons of garbage was stacked up on the streets each day. What stinking filth! When we kill our garbage men (germs) in the human body, we still have the original filth they were trying to consume, plus continual additions, plus the corpses of all the germs we have killed.

This causes the heart to labor, trying to pump the sludge through the system, pulling calcium from wherever it can to help in this extra labor. Then when we are faced with a calcium deficiency we can develop rheumatic fever (causing a rheumatic heart and a weakened body) that may even go into polio, stroke, multiple sclerosis, muscular dystrophy, etc. The rheumatic fever condition leaves a calcium weakness that can lie dormant for years and then with a new loss of calcium at some future date, can develop into one of these maladies.

We want to build the fever as fast as possible with moisture. Dry fever is a killer, causing infantile paralysis, brain fever, etc., but a moist fever can go much higher and if used properly, by working with the germs can only do good as the Maker of this human body intended.

In order to allow skin eruptions to properly be cleansed from the body, we recommend the following version of the Cold Sheet Treatment. This procedure is not as in-depth as the full treatment described in Appendix C, but will suffice to aid the body to cleanse and heal during Chicken Pox, Measles, etc.

To begin with, check for constipation; and if the fever is quite high, use a catnip tea enema. All teas are made with a teaspoon of herb to a cup of boiling distilled water or an ounce of herb to a pint of boiling distilled water. Pour boiling water over herbs, cover and steep in a warm place fifteen to twenty minutes, strain and use after it cools. Never use aluminum or copper cookware use glass, stainless steel or porcelain.

Insert the cooled tea into the rectum and leave in as long as possible. In this way the loose fecal matter will be voided. In addition, use the bowel aid as mentioned before, such as the Lower Bowel Formula detailed in Appendix A.

Next we use water therapy. After the bowels are cleaned out, put the child into a very warm tub of water, as hot as can be tolerated, and leave him in the tub, keeping it hot (very warm) for as long as possible. Give the child lots of very warm yarrow and/or red raspberry leaf tea to drink, while in the tub, to make him sweat a lot. This will bring the poisons to the surface faster. A fast break-out on the skin will shorten the sick period by a number of days.

When it is time to take the child out of the tub, sponge him off with cold water, and, while still damp, without drying the child off, put on night clothes and bundle off into bed. (Dry the head unless a night-cap is used.) The dampness will keep the poisons coming to the surface, generating an artificial fever which will insure the drying out of the clothes by the time the child awakens in the morning.

In the morning, sponge the child off with warm apple cider vinegar and distilled water, mixed half and half. Put him into clean night clothes, change the bed linen and give him some vegetable or fruit juice and let him go back to bed for awhile. When he feels well and energetic enough, let him go back to his activities. Keep him on juice and/or ripe fruit, distilled water, slippery elm gruel, comfrey green drink or comfrey tea.

APPENDIX F

HOW TO MAKE SIMPLE HERBAL PREPARATIONS

Tea. Herbal teas are prepared by using one teaspoonful of the herb to a cup of distilled water or one ounce of herb to the pint of water. Pour the boiling water over the herb, cover tightly and steep for twenty minutes and strain. Sweeten with a little honey, if needed, then give at body temperature or warmer. The dosage is: one cup three times in a day, more or less as needed. Twelve years and up, as above, full adult dose; eight to twelve years, one half adult dose; four to eight years, one fourth; and below four years of age, divide child s weight by 150, and administer the percentage (e.g. 32 lbs = 22% of adult dosage).

Poultice. A poultice is an herbal preparation of a soft, semi-liquid mass made of some cohesive substance mixed with water, apple cider vinegar or other substances, and used for supplying heat and moisture to an area, or to act as a local stimulant. Have the herbs ground or granulated. When using fine powder, just use enough moisture to make a thick paste; and when using the granulated form, a thick paste may be made with a mixture of water and corn meal (or flaxseed meal). If fresh green leaves are used, simply heat, bruise, triturate or chop them up finely, and apply to the affected parts. Poultices are excellent for enlarged or inflamed glands (neck, breast, groin, prostate, etc.), and also for eruptions, boils, carbuncles, and abscesses.

Fomentation. A fomentation is applying herbs to convey heat, moisture, and medicinal aid in order to relieve pain, to reduce inflammation, and to relax affected areas. Fomentations are usually made from bitter herbs, sometimes with cayenne added, steeped in apple cider vinegar or water. A fomentation of apple cider vinegar alone will often take the pain out of arthritis, rheumatism and similar conditions. Soak a Turkish towel or gauze or similar material in the hot herbal tea, lightly wring (just enough that the liquid will not run off the body), and place over the affected area as hot as possible without causing blistering. Generally keep the fomentation moist and warm by placing plastics, oilcloth, etc., over fomentation. Dosage: Wet enough that the moisture will not run off the body, cover entire malfunction area, keep damp and change periodically.

APPENDIX G

HERBAL FORMULAS

Formula Name Changes

Most people familiar with Dr. Christopher s writings will notice that many of the herbal formulas names have changed over the years. They were first given descriptive names such as lung tonic or intestinal tonic. Then, because of government regulations the word tonic was replaced by the word palliative. Soon, laws were passed and the names had to be changed again to non-descriptive aliases such as BF&C or Fen-LB that really didn t let the consumer know what the formulas were used for. The formula labels remained in this encoded and cryptic form for many years. Recently, the rules concerning product names were changed again, this time allowing them to be more descriptive. These new names are easier for the consumer to understand. In this appendix, the most recent names are listed first and the older names are listed in parentheses. This will help those who have older texts and videos relate to these changes.

Comfrey

Another recent development involves the use of comfrey (*Symphytum officinale*). Comfrey has a long track record of safe and effective use as a medicine. It has also been used safely as food for both humans and animals. This aside, comfrey has been the subject of recent controversy. One of the constituents of comfrey is a pyrrolizidine alkaloid that, if taken in large amounts, under certain conditions, may cause liver damage. This is a very rare occurrence and need not concern the average comfrey user. People who need to exercise caution with comfrey are those with chronic liver conditions (such as hepatitis, or cirrhosis) and those who are taking liver compromising medications. Due to new government policy, no herbal product containing comfrey may be sold for internal use. Because of this, some herbal recipes have been re-formulated to include other healing herbs to replace comfrey (bulk formulas with comfrey are still available for external use). The School of Natural Healing maintains that this wonderful healing herb should be available to all who would like to use it, and looks forward to the day that comfrey will be once again be accessible to everyone. In this index, the formulas are listed both in their original form (with comfrey) and with the recent changes.

Kid-e-line

David Christopher has developed a series of herbal remedies for children called the Kid-e-line. Many of these formulas were modeled after Dr. Christopher s formulas but are prepared with glycerine making them more palatable for children. The names of these formulas are listed along with the names of the formulas they were modeled after.

Dosage

Most Christopher formulas are tonics, which means they may be taken for extended periods of time for chronic problems. The normal tonic dosage is two capsules three times a day or ten to thirty drops of extract three times a day. However, when the need arises this amount may be increased. For example, during an acute infection it may be necessary to take two tablespoons of the Super Garlic Immune Formula every hour even though the normal dose is two tablespoons three times a day. Many inexperienced herb users make the mistake of taking too little a dose. There are two considerations when using herbs as medicine. First, be familiar with the herbs you are using and second, the dosage (or therapy) should be more aggressive than the disease being treated.

Christopher Formulas

Adrenal Formula (Adrenetone)

Mullein (*Verbascum thapsus*)
Lobelia (*Lobelia inflata*)
Siberian Ginseng (*Eleutherococcus senticosus*)
Licorice (*Glycyrrhiza glabra*)
Gotu Kola (*Centella asiatica*)
Hawthorn (*Crataegus laevigata*)
Cayenne (*Capsicum spp.*)
Ginger (*Zingiber officinale*)

The adrenals are responsible for the fight or flight response and also help the body maintain a healthy balance of sugar and salt. This formula helps counteract the effects of long-term stress by providing nutrition that supports the adrenal glands.

Anti-Spasmodic Tincture (AntiSp)

Skullcap (*Scutellaria laterifloria*)
Lobelia (*Lobelia inflata*)
Cayenne (*Capsicum spp.*)
Valerian (*Valeriana officinalis*)
Skunk Cabbage (*Symplocarpus foetidus*)
Myrrh Gum (*Commiphora myrrha*)
Black Cohosh (*Cimicifuga racemosa*)

To be used in cases of convulsions, fainting, cramps, delirium, spasming muscles, tremors, and hysteria. This formula is also good for pyorrhea, mouth sores, coughs, throat infections, and tonsillitis.

Appetite Formula (CSK)

Chickweed (*Stellaria media*)
Burdock (*Arctium lappa*)
Licorice (*Glycyrrhiza glabra*)
Safflower (*Carthamus tinctorius*)
Fennel (*Foeniculum vulgare*)
Parsley Root (*Petroselinum crispum*)
Kelp (*Laminaria saccharina* or *Fucus vesiculosis*)

Echinacea (*Echinacea spp.*)
Black Walnut (*Juglans nigra*)
Hawthorn (*Crataegus laevigata*)
Papaya (*Carica papaya*)

Combine this formula with Dr. Christopher s Mucusless Diet for effective and permanent weight loss. The Appetite Formula supports the kidneys, thyroid, and circulatory system, as well as other glands and organs. It is designed to assist the body in losing weight by controlling the appetite. For best results, take throughout the day with chickweed tea or combine with the Metaburn Weight Management Formula.

Aromatic Nose Therapy Ointment (Nose Ointment)

Spearmint essential oil (*Mentha spicata*)
Peppermint essential oil (*Mentha piperita*)
Non-petroleum jelly base

This formula contains essential oils that are natural antihistamines and work to clear up congestion. Apply to the inside of the nose when congested, dry, sensitive or chapped. This formula also works well for chapped lips.

Bee Power Energy Formula (Bee Power)

Bee pollen
Siberian Ginseng (*Eleutherococcus senticosus*)
Licorice (*Glycyrrhiza glabra*)
Gotu Kola (*Centella asiatica*)
Brigham Tea (*Ephedra nevadensis*)
Yerba Mate (*Ilex paraguariensis*)
Ginger (*Zingiber officinale*)

Rather than being an unnatural energy jolt that shocks the body, this formula provides sustained energy and vitality through wholesome nutrition. This formula works well for athletes, scholars, and busy moms and dads.

Bilberry Eye Formula (Billbrite Formula)

Bilberry (*Vaccinium myrtillus*)
Eyebright (*Euphrasia officinalis*)

Ginkgo (*Ginkgo biloba*)
Cayenne (*Capsicum spp.*)

Bilberry fruit was frequently taken during World War II by British pilots to enhance their night vision before flights. This herbal formula contains additional herbs that increase blood circulation to the eyes helping to repair damaged vessels, improve night vision, cleanse ocular tissues, and bring antioxidants to the eyes.

Black Ointment

Chaparral (*Larrea tridentata*)
Comfrey (*Symphytum officinale*)
Red Clover (*Trifolium pratense*)
Pine Tar (*Pinus spp.*)
Mullein (*Verbascum thapsus*)
Lobelia (*Lobelia inflata*)
Goldenseal (*Hydrastis canadensis*)
Marshmallow Root (*Althea officinalis*)
Plantain (*Plantago major*)
Chickweed (*Stellaria media*)
Poke Root (*Phytolacca americana*)
Bee s wax and olive oil base (This formula was originally made with a mutton tallow base. The commercial version of this formula does not contain tallow or any other animal product.)

This formula is for external use on old ulcers, tumors, boils, warts, skin cancers, hemorrhoids, and burns.

Black Walnut Tincture

Black Walnut (*Juglans nigra*)

Black Walnut has been used for centuries to treat fungal infections. It is also helpful in cases of warts or parasitic infections.

Bladder Formula, Kid-e-Dry (DRI formula)

Parsley Root (*Petroselinum crispum*)
Juniper (*Juniperus communis*)
Marshmallow Root (*Althaea officinalis*)
White Pond Lily (*Nymphaea odorata*)

Gravel Root (*Eupatorium purpureum*)
Uva Ursi (*Arctostaphylos uva-ursi*)
Lobelia (*Lobelia inflata*)
Ginger (*Zingiber officinalis*)
Black Cohosh (*Cimicifuga racemosa*)

This formula is a specific for controlling or overcoming incontinence and for strengthening the entire urinary tract including the urethral canal, kidneys, and bladder. Recommended dosage is two No. 0 capsules three times a day with a cup of parsley tea. For bed wetting: upon retiring at night fasten a six or eight inch ball of yarn, string, or cloth onto night clothes in the middle of the back. This prevents the individual from lying on their back, which is generally the position that people void urine.

Blood Circulation Formula (BPE, Blood Pressure Formula)

Ginger (*Zingiber officinalis*)
Cayenne (*Capsicum spp.*)
Goldenseal (*Hydrastis canadensis*)
Siberian Ginseng (*Eleutherococcus senticosus*)
Parsley Root (*Petroselinum crispum*)
Garlic (*Allium sativum*)

This formula is designed to normalize blood pressure throughout the body. It has worked in cases of both low and high blood pressure.

Blood Stream Formula (Red Clover Combination or RCC)

Red Cover Blossoms (*Trifolium pratense*)
Chaparral (*Larrea tridentata*)
Licorice (*Glycyrrhiza glabra*)
Poke Root (*Phytolacca americana*)
Peach Bark (*Prunus persica*)
Oregon Grape (*Mahonia aquifolium; M. repens*)
Stillingia (*Stillingia sylvatica*)
Cascara Sagrada (*Rhamnus purshiana*)
Sarsaparilla (*Smilax officinalis*)
Prickly Ash (*Zanthoxylum americanum*)
Burdock (*Arctium lappa*)

Buckthorn (*Rhamnus frangula*)

The circulatory system plays an important role in the body by delivering food to all the cells and carrying off the waste materials. This herbal blood building formula is designed to help cleanse the blood down to the cellular level. It also aids in removing cholesterol, builds elasticity and strength in veins and artery walls. Some of the herbs contained in this formula are potent infection fighters.

Breathe-Free

Brigham Tea (*Ephedra nevadensis*)
Horseradish (*Armoracia rusticana*)
Marshmallow Root (*Althea officinalis*)
Cayenne (*Capsicum spp.*)
Garlic (*Allium sativum*)
Rose Hips (*Rosa spp.*)
Watercress (*Nasturtium officinale*)
Feverfew (*Tanacetum parthenium*)

This formula is a natural decongestant, soothes irritated lung tissue, eases pain and tension, and inhibits bacterial growth.

Cayenne Heating Balm (Deep Heating Balm or Cayenne Salve)

Cayenne (*Capsicum spp.*)
Wintergreen essential oil (*Gaultheria procumbens*)
Pure distilled mint crystals and other herbal oils
Beeswax and olive oil base

This penetrating salve is excellent for stiff necks, sore muscles, headaches, muscular pain, stiff joints, arthritis, etc. The Cayenne Heating Balm can be used with other ointments, creams, and salves as a catalyst, driving their healing power deeper into the body.

Chest Formula (Herbal Composition Powder)

Bayberry (*Berberis vulgaris*)
Cloves (*Syzygium aromaticum*)
Ginger (*Zingiber officinale*)
Cayenne (*Capsicum spp.*)
White Pine (*Pinus strobus*)

Dr. Nowell, one of Dr. Christopher s instructors at the Dominion Herbal College of Vancouver, B.C. had this to say about the Chest Formula, W e have made and used composition powder for over forty years. When we state we regularly mixed it in batches of sixty pounds, the student will readily see that we have had at least some experience with it. As a remedy in colds, beginning of fevers, flu, hoarseness, sluggish circulation, colic, cramps, etc., we believe it has done more good than any other single preparation ever known to man. If this compound were kept in every home, and used as the occasion arose, there would be far less sickness. Give it freely in your practice and your patient will bless you. Look over the ingredients and consider how it will clear canker, ease cramps and pains in the stomach and bowels, raise the heat of the body equalizing the circulation, and removing congestions. It is safe. It is effective. We have on numberless occasions given a cup of composition tea every hour, as warm as the patient could drink it, until the patient has perspired freely, and after four or five doses , we have seen our patients in a free perspiration, thereby removing colds and febrile trouble.

Cold Season Formula (GR&P or Garlic, Rose hips, and Parsley)

Garlic (*Allium sativum*)
Parsley Root (*Petroselinum crispum*)
Watercress (*Nasturtium officinale*)
Rosemary (*Rosmarinus officinalis*)
Rose Hips (*Rosa spp.*)

This herbal formula is designed to support the immune system. It consists of some of the top sources of natural anti-oxidants. It may be taken regularly during flu and cold season.

Cold Sore Relief (CSR)

Goldenseal (*Hydrastis canadensis*)
Garlic (*Allium sativum*)
Skullcap (*Scutellaria lateriflloria*)

Cold sores are not only a nuisance, but can be extremely contagious. This herbal formula addresses the cause of cold sores and stops them from recurring.

Complete Tissue and Bone Formula (BF&C)

White Oak (*Quercus alba*)
Marshmallow Root (*Althea officinalis*)
Mullein (*Verbascum thapsus*)
Wormwood (*Artemisia absinthium*)
Lobelia (*Lobelia inflata*)
Skullcap (*Scutellaria laterifloria*)
Comfrey (*Symphytum officinale*)
Replaced with Lungwort (*Pulmonaria officinalis*), Slippery Elm (*Ulmus rubra*), and Plantain (*Plantago major*)
Black Walnut (*Juglans nigra*)
Gravel Root (*Eupatorium purpureum*)

This formula is an aid for malfunction in bone, flesh, and cartilage. It has been used to treat broken bones, sprained ankles, torn ligaments, scrapes, cuts, and wounds. It is also excellent for varicose veins, curvature of the spine, skin eruptions, pulled muscles, blood clots, and calcium spurs. It may be used in capsules, tea, syrup, fomentation, ointment, oil, cream, or poultice.

Cycle-Eze

Blessed Thistle (*Cnicus benedictus*)
Dong Quai (*Angelica sinensis*)
Bupleurum (*Bupleurum chinensis*)
Squawvine (*Mitchella repens*)
Red Clover (*Trifolium pratense*)
Cramp Bark (*Viburnum opulus*)
Black Cohosh (*Cimicifuga racemosa*)
Sarsaparilla (*Smilax medica*)
Uva ursi (*Arctostaphylos uva ursi*)
Marshmallow (*Althea officinalis*)

This formula is used is to aid the body during times of bloating, pain and general discomfort, as well as to promote normal menstruation while tonifying the entire female body.

Ear and Nerve Formula (B&B Glycerine Extract)

Blue Cohosh (*Caulophyllum thalictroides*)
Black Cohosh (*Cimicifuga racemosa*)
Blue Vervain (*Verbena hastata*)
Skullcap (*Scutellaria lateriflora*)
Lobelia (*Lobelia inflata*)

This formula has been used to improve poor equilibrium, reverse hearing loss, and to heal malfunctioning nerves (tinnitus). The procedure is as follows: Place four to six drops of oil of garlic and four to six drops of this formula in each ear before bed. Plug the ears overnight with cotton, six days a week, for four to six months, or as needed. On the seventh day, flush ears with an ear syringe using half warm apple cider vinegar and half distilled water. In cases of a ruptured ear drum, do not use apple cider vinegar.

False Unicorn and Lobelia Formula (Anti-Miscarriage Formula)

False Unicorn (*Chamaelirium luteum*)
Lobelia (*Lobelia inflata*)

If hemorrhaging starts during pregnancy, stay in bed, use a bed pan when needed, and use ß cup of the tea (or two #0 capsules) each ß hour until bleeding stops, then each waking hour for one day. After the first day, continue taking two capsules of this formula three times a day for three weeks, staying in bed as much as possible. If bleeding continues instead of decreasing, see a qualified health care professional. This formula has also been used (two capsules three times a day) to treat infertility.

Female Reproductive Formula (Nu-Fem)

Goldenseal (*Hydrastis canadensis*)
Blessed Thistle (*Cnicus benedictus*)
Cayenne (*Capsicum spp.*)
Cramp Bark (*Viburnum opulus*)
False Unicorn (*Chamaelirium luteum*)
Ginger (*Zingiber officinale*)
Red Raspberry (*Rubus idaeus*)
Squawvine (*Mitchella Repens*)

Uva Ursi (*Arctostaphylos uva ursi*)

This is an amazing herbal formula which was designed to aid in rebuilding a malfunctioning female reproductive system (uterus, ovaries, fallopian tubes, etc.). Over the years herbalists and patients have seen painful menstruation, heavy flowing, cramps, irregularity, and inability to conceive, change to a painless menstrual period, good menstrual timing, and a new outlook on life by using this herbal aid to readjust the malfunctioning organs. We have seen many people with severe cases that have had years of suffering cleared up in 90 to 120 days. Some get relief sooner, some take longer no two cases are alike.

Female Tonic Formula (Fematone)

Squawvine (*Mitchella repens*)
Red Raspberry (*Rubus idaeus*)
Nettle (*Urtica dioica*)
Dandelion (*Taraxacum officinale*)
Wild Yam (*Dioscorea villosa*)
Cramp Bark (*Viburnum opulus*)
Chickweed (*Stellaria media*)
Purple Dulse (*Rhodymenia palmetta*)
Vitex (*Vitex agnus castus*)
Motherwort (*Leonurus cardiaca*)
Ginger (*Zingiber officinale*)

This formula is designed to strengthen and nourish the female reproductive organs. It is a tonic formula that may be taken daily for an extended period of time.

Gas-Eze

Cayenne (*Capsicum spp.*)
Papain Enzyme (*Carica papaya*)
Slippery Elm (*Ulmus rubra*)
Caraway Seed (*Carum carvi*)
Ginger (*Zingiber officinale*)
Catnip (*Nepeta cataria*)

This formula stimulates the digestive process, neutralizes stomach acidity and soothes and protects the entire digestive system.

Glandular System Formula (Mullein and Lobelia Formula)

Mullein (*Verbascum thapsus*)
Lobelia (*Lobelia inflata*)

This herbal formula works by cleansing and nourishing the glands and lymph organs of the body. It may be used in capsules, ointment, oil, or as a fomentation. It is best to use this formula in conjunction with lymph stimulating exercise (jump rope or trampoline) to encourage lymph to flow throughout the body.

Hawthorn Berry Heart Syrup (Hawthorn Berry Syrup)

Hawthorn Berry (*Crataegus oxycantha*)
Glycerine and grape brandy base

Hawthorn has been used for centuries as a food for the heart. *Potter s Cyclopaedia of Botanical Drugs and Preparations*, (an old English herbals) lists hawthorn as a cardiac tonic. Hawthorn has been used to treat functional heart disorders such as dyspnoea, rapid and feeble heart action, hypertrophy, valvular insufficiency, and heart oppression.

Heavy Mineral Bugleweed Formula (Bugledock Combination)

Bugleweed (*Lycopus Virginicus*)
Yellow Dock (*Rumex crispus*)
Lobelia (*Lobelia inflata*)
Cilantro (*Coriandrum sativum*) added in 2001

This herbal formula is designed to help the body rid itself of toxic contamination. It helps draw out minerals, drugs, and other pollutants trapped in the body. The dosage is two #0 capsules daily in conjunction with six #0 chaparral capsules taken three times a day. (This formula including the chaparral, is available in extract form.) Every other day bathe in an Epsom salt bath (add one to three pounds of Epsom salts in a tub of hot water). This bathing routine should continue for three weeks, allowing the body to rest one week before continuing with more Epsom salt baths if necessary. The cilantro in this formula (which was added to the formula in 2001) was added specifically to draw mercury accumulations out of the body.

Herbalert

Gotu Kola (*Centella asiatica*)
Blue Vervain (*Verbena hastata*)
Brigham Tea (*Ephedra nevadensis*)
Yerba Mate (*Ilex paraguariensis*)
Blessed Thistle (*Cnicus benedictus*)
Mullein (*Verbascum thapsus*)
Siberian Ginseng (*Eleutherococcus senticosus*)
Cayenne (*Capsicum spp.*)
Ginger (*Zingiber officinalis*)
Shizandra (*Shizandra chinensis*)
Garlic (*Allium sativum*)

Herbalert assists the body in overcoming stress and helps normalize hormones and blood sugar levels. It also stimulates circulation to the brain, soothing and toning the central nervous system, while supplying extra energy.

Herbal Bolus (VB Combination)

Squawvine (*Mitchella repens*)
Slippery Elm (*Ulmus rubra*)
Yellow Dock (*Rumex crispus*)
Comfrey (*Symphytum officinale*)
Marshmallow Root (*Althea officinalis*)
Chickweed (*Stellaria media*)
Goldenseal (*Hydrastis canadensis*)
Mullein (*Verbascum thapsus*)

Here is another excellent aid for both men and women who have problems in their reproductive organs. Boluses are made with healing herbs that feed malnourished organs and draw out toxic accumulations, making the malfunctioning area clean and healthy. Herbalists who use this formula have found it helpful in cases of tumors, cysts, and lesions in the reproductive organs. The bolus spreads its herbal influence widely from the vagina or bowel through the urinary and genital organs. To make a bolus with this formula, melt coconut butter so that it will mix well with the herb powder. Mix a small quantity of this formula with coconut butter until the consistency of pie dough is achieved. Next, roll this mass with your hands until you have a pencil-like bolus approximately the size of the middle finger, cut in inch-long lengths. Harden the bolus in a refrigerator for a few hours. These are to be inserted into the vagina or rectum much the same as a suppository would be. It may be necessary to wear a sanitary napkin so as not to soil clothing when the bolus is melted. Insert upon retiring and leave in all night, six nights a week. The coconut butter melts at body temperature, leaving only the herbs, which are absorbed by the body. On the seventh morning use the Iron Assimilation Formula as a douche to wash out any remaining material.

Herbal Calcium Formula, Kid-e-Calc (Calc-Tea)

Horsetail (*Equisetum hyemale*)
Oat Straw (*Avena sativa*)
Comfrey (*Symphytum officinale*)
Replaced with Nettle (*Urtica dioica*)
Lobelia (*Lobelia inflata*)

We need calcium in our bodies for many purposes, for a healthy nerve sheath, healthy vein and artery walls, strong bones, and healthy teeth. This herbal formula provides calcium along with silica and other nutrients that support calcium absorption. It may also be used for cramps, charlie horses, jumping leg syndrome, children with crooked teeth, teething problems, a healthy pregnancy, and all other calcium needs in the body. As explained earlier, comfrey was recently taken out of many of the formulas. In this formula, comfrey was replaced by nettles, which have a high amount of natural calcium.

Herbal Eyebright Formula (Herbal Eye Wash Formula)

Bayberry Bark (*Berberis vulgaris*)
Eyebright (*Euphrasia officinalis*)
Goldenseal (*Hydrastis canadensis*)
Red Raspberry (*Rubus idaeus*)
Cayenne (*Capsicum spp.*)

This formula is excellent for brightening and healing the eyes, and is known to remove cataracts and heavy film. It has also been used to correct vision problems including near sightedness, far sightedness, macular degeneration, and glaucoma. There will be a burning sensation when using the eyewash at first. This is due to the stimulating effect of the cayenne pepper and will do nothing but good for the eyes. Directions: When using the tincture, add two to five drops of the extract in an eyecup of boiled water. Let the solution cool to body temperature and wash the eye by holding the eyecup to the eye and tipping the head backwards. Exercise the eye while doing this as though you were swimming. Be sure to use a different eyecup for each eye so there is no cross-contamination if infection is present. Do this three to six times a day and take two capsules or a cup of the tea, morning and evening.

Herbal Cough Syrup

Wild Cherry (*Prunus serotina*)
Licorice (*Glycyrrhiza glabra*)
Marshmallow Root (*Althea officinalis*)
Horehound (*Marrubium vulgare*)
Mullein (*Verbascum thapsus*)
Ginger (*Zingiber officinale*)
Anise (*Pempinella anisum*)
Lemon Peel (*Citrus limon*)

This formula reduces mucus buildup and acts as an anti-biotic, while soothing the throat. This formula is especially useful for dry, scratchy throats.

Herbal Iron Formula (Prolapse Formula, Yellow Dock Combination)

Oak Bark (*Quercus alba*)
Mullein (*Verbascum thapsus*)
Yellow Dock (*Rumex crispus*)
Black Walnut (*Juglans nigra*)
Comfrey (*Symphytum officinale*)
 Replaced with Slippery Elm (*Ulmus rubra*) and
 Plantain (*Plantago major*)
Lobelia (*Lobelia inflata*)
Marshmallow Root (*Althea officinalis*)

To build and relieve prolapsed uterus, bowel, or other organs or for hemorrhoid problems, make a concentrated tea of this formula (simmer down to half its amount). Inject with a syringe (while head down on a slant board) into vagina or rectum, 1/4 to 1/2 cup. Leave in as long as possible before voiding. During this procedure, knead and massage the pelvic and abdominal area to exercise muscles so the herbal tea (food) will be assimilated into the organs. It is helpful to drink 1/4 cup of tea concentrate in 3/4 cup of distilled water three times a day or take two capsules three times a day.

Herbal Parasite Syrup (VF Syrup)

Wormwood (*Artemisia absinthium*)
American Wormseed (*Chenopodium anthelminticum*)
Garden Sage (*Salvia officinalis*)
Fennel (*Foeniculum vulgare*)
Male Fern (*Dryopteris filix-mas*)
Papaya (*Carica papaya*)

This formula acts as a vermifuge (herbal agent that will cause expulsion of worms from the body) and/or vermicide (herbal agent that destroys worms in the body). Recommended dosage is one teaspoon each morning and night for three days. On the fourth day drink one cup of senna and peppermint tea, using ß teaspoon of each in a cup of hot, distilled water. Rest two days and repeat two more times.

Herbal Thyroid Formula (Thyroid Stimulating Formula)

Guarana (*Paullinia cupana*)
Siberian Ginseng (*Eleutherococcus senticosus*)
Fo-Ti (*Polygonum multiflorum*)
Gotu Kola (*Centella asiatica*)
Mullein (*Verbascum thapsus*)
Kelp (*Ascophyllum nodosum*)

This formula stimulates the underactive thyroid, but is not intended for long term use. Use this formula for a month and then switch to the Thyroid Maintenance Formula which may be used for a longer period of time.

Herbal Tooth and Gum Powder (Herbal Tooth Powder)

Oak Bark (*Quercus alba*)

Comfrey (*Symphytum officinale*)
Replaced with Stevia (*Stevia rebaudiana*), Bayberry (*Berberis vulgaris*), and Slippery Elm (*Ulmus rubra*)
Horsetail (*Equisetum hyemale*)
Lobelia (*Lobelia inflata*)
Replaced with Prickly Ash (*Zanthoxylum americanum*)
Cloves (*Syzygium aromaticum*)
Peppermint (*Mentha piperita*)

This formula is designed to help strengthen gums and assist in tightening loose teeth. The tooth powder will brighten tooth luster and make for a healthier mouth as well as fight infections. For severe cases, place this herbal formula between the lips and gums (upper and lower) around entire tooth area and leave on all night, six nights a week (as well as brushing regularly) until improvement is evident. Then continue on with regular brushing with this herbal formula. When packing the gums overnight, mix this tooth powder with extra slippery elm. The recent changes to this formula have made it more palatable and easier to use.

Hormonal Changease (Changease)
Black Cohosh (*Cimicifuga racemosa*)
Sarsaparilla (*Smilax medica*)
Siberian Ginseng (*Eleutherococcus senticosus*)
Licorice (*Glycyrrhiza glabra*)
False Unicorn (*Chamaelirium luteum*)
Blessed Thistle (*Cnicus benedictus*)
Squawvine (*Mitchella repens*)

This is an herbal food designed to provide the building blocks needed to create and maintain proper hormone levels. Hormone levels rise and fall at different stages of life including adolescence, pre-natal, post-natal, and menopause. Women and men both experience hormonal changes throughout life and this formula assists the body as it adjusts to new hormone levels.

Immucalm, Kid-e-Soothe
Marshmallow Root (*Althea officinalis*)

Astragalus (*Astragalus membranaceus*)

This formula is designed to calm yet strengthen the body s immune response. Signs of an overactive immune system include: allergic reactions to certain foods, plants, or animals, or auto-immune diseases. This simple combination of marshmallow root and astragalus has made life easier for those who suffer from allergies, hay fever, asthma, multiple sclerosis, juvenile onset diabetes, rheumatoid arthritis, or any hyperactive immune response. This formula also stimulates the body s ability to fight off infection.

Immune System Formula (Immutone):

Astragalus (*Astragalus membranaceus*)
Siberian Ginseng (*Eleutherococcus senticosus*)
Echinacea (*Echinacea spp.*)
Reishi Mushroom (*Ganoderma lucidum*)

This tonic formula helps strengthen the immune system and guard against invaders. This formula is very effective when taken at the first signs of sickness to stop it in its tracks.

Itch Ointment (Chickweed Ointment)

Chickweed (*Stellaria media*)
Bee s wax and olive oil base

This is a wonderful healing ointment for eczema, sores, psoriasis, burning, itchy skin or genitals, swollen testes, acne, and hives.

Joint Formula (AR-1)

Brigham Tea (*Ephedra nevadensis*)
Hydrangea (*Hydrangea arborescens*)
Yucca (*Yucca schidigera*)
Chaparral (*Larrea tridentata*)
Lobelia (*Lobelia inflata*)
Burdock (*Actium lappa*)
Sarsaparilla (*Smilax medica*)
Wild Lettuce (*Lactuca spp.*)
Valerian (*Valeriana officinalis*)
Wormwood (*Artemisia tridentata*)

Cayenne (*Capsicum spp.*)
Black Cohosh (*Cimicifuga racemosa*)
Black Walnut (*Juglans nigra*)

Arthritis and joint pain have many different causes. This formula acts as an anti-inflammatory, cleanses the blood, eases pain, and addresses the hormonal aspects of joint pain.

Jurassic Green

Alfalfa (*Medicago sativa*)
Barley Grass (*Hordeum vulgare*)
Wheat Grass (*Triticum spp.*)

This herbal food is made from herbs grown organically in virgin soil and separated from urban and agricultural pollutants by the same mountains that provide its pure source of water. These herbs reduce acidity, provide needed chlorophyll and wholesome nutrients to the body. With the proper ingredients the body is then able to produce blood, make hormones, and has the building blocks needed to heal injured tissue. Jurassic Green comes in a powder that may be mixed with water or any fruit or vegetable juice.

Kid-e-Calc (Glycerine form of the Herbal Calcium Formula with natural flavoring)

Kid-e-Col (Glycerine form of the Catnip and Fennel Formula with natural favoring)

Kid-e-Dry (Glycerine form of the Bladder Formula with natural flavoring)

Kid-e-Mins (Glycerine form of the Vitalerbs Formula with natural flavoring)

Kid-e-Mune

Echinacea (*Echinacea spp.*)
Glycerine base with natural flavoring

This formula is designed to enhance the body s ability to prevent and fight the spread of bacteria and viruses.

Kid-e-Reg

Slippery Elm (*Ulmus rubra*)
Fennel (*Foeniculum vulgare*)
Licorice (*Glycyrrhiza glabra*)
Anise (*Pempinella anisum*)
Fig Syrup (*Ficus carica*)
Glycerine base

This gentle bowel formula supports the intestines and acts as mild laxative. It is safe to use for an extended period of time if needed.

Kid-e-Soothe (Glycerine form of the Immucalm Formula with natural flavoring)

Kid-e-Trac (Glycerine form of the MindTrac Formula with natural flavoring)

Kid-e-Well

Yarrow (*Achillea millefolium*)
Elder (*Sambucus nigra*)
Peppermint (*Mentha piperita*)
Echinacea (*Echinacea angustifolia*)

This formula is mildly stimulating to the immune system. It allows your child to naturally combat colds and flu, and fever. It is a great aid for relaxing and calming the nerves during the healing process.

Kidney Formula (Juni-Pars)

Juniper (*Juniperus communis*)
Parsley (*Petroselinum crispum*)
Uva Ursi (*Arctostaphylos uva-ursi*)
Marshmallow Root (*Althaea officinalis*)
Lobelia (*Lobelia inflata*)
Ginger (*Zingiber officinalis*)
Goldenseal (*Hydrastis canadensis*)

Approximately eighty percentage of the body is liquid and much of this fluid must be pumped, filtered, etc., through the body s urinary system. We generally do not take the best care of this delicate tract. We ask it to filter hundreds of gallons of hard water, milk, carbonated beverages, and other liquids each year. The result is malfunctioning kidneys, stones, and lower back pain. The Kidney Formula provides specific nutrition for the kidneys and bladder, cleans out deposits, and strengthens the urinary tract walls and muscles. The Kidney Formula is also useful for those with bladder incontinence. For added benefit, use this formula in conjunction with parsley tea.

Liver and Gall Bladder Formula (Barberry LG)

Barberry (*Berberis vulgaris*) or Oregon Grape Root (*Mahonia aquifolium*)
Wild Yam (*Dioscorea villosa*)
Cramp Bark (*Viburnum trilobum; V. opulus*)
Fennel (*Foeniculum vulgare*)
Ginger (*Zingiber officinalis*)
Catnip (*Nepeta cataria*)
Peppermint (*Mentha piperita*)

The liver has numerous functions in the body. One of its main jobs is to filter the blood as it travels throughout the circulatory system. When the liver is not functioning properly, many conditions may result including acne, eczema, hormonal problems, manic depression, anxiety disorder, depression, loss of libido, constipation, cholemia, indigestion, sluggishness, fatigue, upset stomach, chills, vomiting, and fever. The Liver and Gall Bladder Formula supports the proper function of both the liver and gall bladder and helps rebuild and cleanse these organs when necessary.

Liver Transition Formula (PreTrac)

Siberian Ginseng (*Eleutherococcus senticosus*)
Rosemary (*Rosmarinus officinalis*)
Ginkgo (*Ginkgo biloba*)
Oregon Grape Root (*Mahonia aquifolium*)
Milk Thistle (*Silybum marianum*)
Wild Yam (*Dioscorea villosa*)
Skullcap (*Scutellaria lateriflora*)

Jurassic Green

This formula assists the body during the transition from psychiatric drugs to herbal supplements. It gently cleanses the liver, provides energy and stamina, and addresses both hormonal and nervous aspects of depression. Because of the seriousness of some emotional conditions, and the side-effects of most psychiatric drugs, it is necessary to seek advice from a qualified health care provider before attempting to wean oneself off of these medications.

Lower Bowel Formula (Fen LB or Herbal LB)

Barberry (*Berberis vulgaris*)
Cascara Sagrada (*Rhamnus purshiana*)
Cayenne (*Capsicum spp.*)
Ginger (*Zingiber officinale*)
Lobelia (*Lobelia inflata*)
Red Raspberry (*Rubus idaeus*)
Turkey Rhubarb (*Rheum palmatum*)
Fennel (*Foeniculum vulgaris*)
Goldenseal (*Hydrastis canadensis*)

After years of working with people all over the country, Dr. Christopher noticed that well over ninety-five percent off all disease is caused by constipation. When his patients used the Lower Bowel Formula and changed their diet, they regained health and their diseases were cured and didn t come back. This formula is not a simple herbal laxative, The Lower Bowel Formula re-builds the tissues of the colon and strengthens intestinal muscles. For more information on intestinal health see *Dr. Christopher s Guide to Colon Health* published by Christopher Publications.

Lung and Bronchial Formula (Resp-Free)

Comfrey (*Symphytum officinale*)
Replaced with Pleurisy Root (*Asclepias tuberose*)
Mullein (*Verbascum thapsus*)
Chickweed (*Stellaria media*)
Marshmallow Root (*Althaea officinalis*)
Lobelia (*Lobelia inflata*)

This formula is extremely valuable in strengthening and healing the entire respiratory tract. It promotes the discharge of mucus secretions from the bronchio-pulmonary passages and relieves irritation in the respiratory tract, lungs and bronchials. It has been useful in cases of emphysema as well as bronchitis, asthma, and tuberculosis. For additional help it may be necessary to add three to six drops of tincture of lobelia to each dose.

Lymphatic Formula (INF Combination)

Plantain (*Plantago major*)
Black Walnut (*Juglans nigra*)
Goldenseal (*Hydrastis canadensis*)
Bugleweed (*Lycopus virginicus*)
Marshmallow Root (*Althea officinalis*)
Lobelia (*Lobelia inflata*)

This wonderful formula kills infection and clears toxins from the lymph system.

Male Tonic Formula (Mascutone)

Siberian Ginseng (*Eleutherococcus senticosus*)
Sarsaparilla (*Smilax medica*)
Red Raspberry (*Rubus idaeus*)
Saw Palmetto (*Serenoa repens*)
Ginkgo (*Gingko biloba*)
Pumpkin Seeds (*Cucurbita pepo*)
Damiana (*Turnera diffusa*)
Bee Pollen
Hops (*Humulus lupulus*)
Dandelion (*Taraxacum officinale*)
Hawthorn (*Crataegus laevigata*)
Cayenne (*Capsicum spp.*)

This formula is an herbal tonic designed to assist in strengthening the male body. Because it is a tonic formula it may be taken for extended periods of time without harm. It supports the proper function of the prostate and reproductive organs, male potency, and circulatory system.

Male Urinary Tract Formula (Prospallate)

Cayenne (*Capsicum spp.*)
Ginger (*Zingiber officinale*)
Goldenseal (*Hydrastis canadensis*)
Gravel Root or Queen of the Meadow (*Eupatorium purpureum*)
Juniper (*Juniperus communis*)
Marshmallow Root (*Althea officinalis*)
Parsley Root or Herb (*Petroselinum crispum*)
Uva Ursi (*Arctostaphylos uva ursi*)
Siberian Ginseng (*Eleutherococcus senticosus*)

This formula helps the body dissolve stones that are in the kidneys, as well as clean out other sedimentation and infection contributing to prostate enlargement.

Master Gland Formula (Master GL)

Carrot Leaf (*Daucus carota*)
Gotu Kola (*Centella asiatica*)
Ginkgo (*Ginkgo biloba*)
Mullein (*Verbascum thapsus*)
Oregon Grape (*Mahonia aquifolium*)
Lobelia (*Lobelia inflata*)

The pituitary (located at the base of the brain) is known as the master gland. It secretes hormones that regulate many body processes including growth, reproduction, and various metabolic activities. When the pituitary gland malfunctions, it may cause growth problems (both dwarfism and gigantism), obesity, and diabetes. This formula supports the pituitary gland so it may function properly.

Memory Plus Formula (MEM Formula)

Blue Vervain (*Verbena hastata*)
Gotu Kola (*Centella asiatica*)
Brigham Tea (*Ephedra nevadensis*)
Ginkgo (*Ginkgo biloba*)
Blessed Thistle (*Cnicus benedictus*)
Cayenne (*Capsicum spp.*)

Ginger (*Zingiber officinale*)
Lobelia (*Lobelia inflata*)

This is a great herbal formula used to cleanse, re-build and increase circulation in the brain.

Metaburn Weight Formula (Metaburn)

Brigham Tea (*Ephedra nevadensis*)
Red Clover (*Trifolium pratense*)
Oat Straw (*Avena sativum*)
Damiana (*Turnera diffusa*)
Chickweed (*Stellaria media*)
Juniper (*Juniperus communis*)
Catnip (*Nepeta cataria*)
Senna (*Senna alexandrina*)
Cayenne (*Capsicum spp.*)

This formula encourages the body to burn calories, and control appetite and hunger pains.

MindTrac, Kid-e-Trac

Valerian (*Valeriana officinalis*)
Skullcap (*Scutellaria laterifloria*)
Ginkgo (*Ginkgo biloba*)
Oregon Grape (*Mahonia repens*)
St. John s Wort (Hypericum perforatum)
Mullein (*Verbascum thapsus*)
Gotu Kola (*Centella asiatica*)
Sarsaparilla (*Smilax medica*)
Dandelion (*Taraxacum officinale*)
Lobelia (*Lobelia inflata*)
Jurassic Green

Today, more than ever, many of us seem to be overwhelmed by the complexities of life. We find that conditions such as mental fatigue, depression, hyperactivity, attention deficit disorder (ADD), and anxiety are driving even the health conscious to seek quick fixes from drugs. The newest of these quick-fix drugs, S.S.R.I. s (Specific Serotonin Re-uptake Inhibitors), used over time, will damage the liver, imbalance body chemicals, and eventually cause depression anxiety and ADD, the very symptoms they were designed to counter. This herbal formula works on the cause of these mental disruptions and effectively restores good health and mental clarity.

Nerve Formula (B&B Alcohol Tincture)

Black Cohosh (*Cimicifuga racemosa*)
Blue Cohosh (*Caulophyllum thalictroides*)
Blue Vervain (*Verbena hastata*)
Skullcap (*Scutellaria laterifloria*)
Lobelia (*Lobelia inflata*)

This herbal formula is used to aid nervous conditions, sore throat, hiccups, restore malfunctioning motor nerves, adjust poor equilibrium and hearing, and is a great blessing to epileptics and those with Tourette s syndrome. Massage into the medulla (base of skull), and upper cervicals, and take two droppersfull in a little water or juice three times a day.

Pancreas Formula (Panc-Tea)

Goldenseal (*Hydrastis canadensis*)
Uva Ursi (*Arctostaphylos uva-ursi*)
Cayenne (*Capsicum spp.*)
Cedar Berries (*Juniperus monosperma*)
Licorice (*Glycyrrhiza glabra*)
Mullein (*Verbascum thapsus*)

This formula supports the proper function of the pancreas. Combined with the proper diet it has been useful in cases of diabetes (Types I and II), hypoglycemia, and other related diseases.

Prenatal Formula

Squawvine (*Mitchella repens*)
Blessed Thistle (*Cnicus benedictus*)
Black Cohosh (*Cimicifuga racemosa*)
Pennyroyal (*Mentha pulegium*)
False Unicorn (*Chamaelirium luteum*)
Red Raspberry(*Rubus idaeus*)

Lobelia (*Lobelia inflata*)

This tea (or two or three capsules) morning and evening is an aid in giving elasticity to the pelvic and vaginal area and strengthening the reproductive organs for easier delivery. The formula should be used only in the last six weeks before time of birth as follows: One capsule per day the first week, two capsules per day the second week and two capsules three times a day from the third week on. Six capsules a day is the maximum dosage suggested.

Prostate Plus Formula (Prospalmetto)

Saw Palmetto (*Serenoa repens*)

Mullein (*Verbascum thapsus*)

Ginkgo (*Ginkgo biloba*)

The Prostate Plus Formula assists the body in reducing swelling of the prostate gland. It also helps to strengthen and tone the prostate while cleansing it with nourishing anti-oxidants.

Quick Colon Formula #1 (Intestinal Corrective Formula #1)

Curacao and Cape Aloes (*Aloe vera*)

Senna (*Senna alexandrina*)

Cascara Sagrada (*Rhamnus purshiana*)

Barberry (*Berberis vulgaris*)

Ginger (*Zingiber officinale*)

Garlic (*Allium sativum*)

African Bird Pepper or Cayenne Pepper (*Capsicum spp.*)

This blend of herbs is a powerful laxative or purgative and was formulated for cases of extreme constipation. Because this formula is a pure laxative and does not feed the bowel, it is not intended for long term use. The normal dosage of this formula starts at one capsule once a day. The dosage increases one capsule each day until the desired results are achieved (two or three bowel movements a day). After these results are achieved, gradually switch to the Lower Bowel Formula for long term maintenance as needed.

Quick Colon Formula #2 (Intestinal Corrective Formula #2)

Flax Seed (*Linum usitatissimum*)
Apple Fruit Pectin (*Malus spp.*)
Bentonite Clay
Psyllium (*Plantago ovata, P. ispaghula*)
Slippery Elm (*Ulmus rubra*)
Marshmallow Root (*Althea officinalis*)
Fennel (*Foeniculum vulgare*)
Activated Willow Charcoal

If a deeper colon cleanse is needed, this formula can be used in conjunction with Quick Colon Formula #1. This formula was designed to pull toxins and deposits out of the colon and eliminate them from the body. This formula is slightly constipating and should not be taken without Quick Colon Formula #1. Also, because of the cleansing nature of this formula, it should be taken with large amounts of water and only when the bowels are regular (two or three bowel movements a day). Directions: Mix one heaping teaspoon of powder with four to six ounces of fresh juice or water. After consumption, drink an additional eight or sixteen ounces of liquid (preferably water). Repeat five times a day until finished with the bottle. The Quick Colon Formula #2 is not intended for long term use.

Rash Formula (CMM Ointment)

Comfrey (*Symphytum officinale*)
Marshmallow Root (*Althea officinalis*)
Calendula (*Calendula officinalis*)
Bee s wax and olive oil base

This is a soothing ointment to be used on lesions, eczema, dry skin, poison ivy, abrasions, burns, hemorrhoids, bruises and swellings.

Relax-Eze

Black Cohosh (*Cimicifuga racemosa*)
Capsicum (*Capsicum spp.*)
Hops (*Humulus lupulus*)
Lobelia (*Lobelia inflata*)
Skullcap (*Scutellaria lateriflora*)

Valerian (*Valeriana officinalis*)
Wood Betony (*Stachys officinalis*)
Mistletoe (*Viscum album*)

This formula contains herbs that feed and revitalize the motor nerve at the base of the skull and help rebuild or feed the spinal cord. This formula is designed to rebuild the frayed nerve sheath, the nerve itself, and its capillaries. Relax-Eze has been used with great success for well over thirty years for relieving nervous tension and insomnia. It is mildly stimulating and yet lessens the irritability and excitement of the nervous system and also helps reduce pain.

Respiratory Syrup (Comfrey Mullein and Garlic, CMG Syrup)
Comfrey (*Symphytum officinale*)
Replaced with Onion (*Allium cepa*), Fennel (*Foeniculum vulgare*), Chickweed (*Stellaria media*), and Nettle (*Urtica dioica*)
Mullein (*Verbascum thapsus*)
Garlic (*Allium sativum*)
Glycerine and apple cider vinegar base

This formula is an excellent asthma and cough remedy. It works by expelling mucus from the respiratory system and fighting infection. Unlike cough syrups that suppress expectoration, this formula acts as an expectorant, helping the body rid itself of mucous build-up.

Sen Sei Menthol Rub Ointment (Sen Sei Balm)
Cassia essential oil (*Cinnamomum cassia*)
Eucalyptus essential oil (*Eucalyptus globulus*)
Cajeput essential oil (*Melaleuca minor*)
Pure menthol essential oil (Gaultheria procumbens)
Camphor crystals (*Cinnamomum camphora*)
Other fragrant natural oil
Bee s wax and olive oil base

This balm brings circulation to the surface of the skin causing it to turn red. It is a great remedy for tension headaches, sinus pressure, and sore muscles. Use sparingly as this formula is strong.

Sinus and Lung Formula (Ephedratean)

Brigham Tea (*Ephedra nevadensis*)
Horseradish (*Armoracia rusticana*)
Cayenne (*Capsicum spp.*)

Use this formula for immediate relief of sinus pressure due to cold or allergies. It stimulates the body to rid itself of mucus and helps relieve pain associated with sinus congestion.

Sinus Plus Formula (SHA-Tea and Sinutean)

Brigham Tea (*Ephedra nevadensis*)
Marshmalow Root (*Althaea officinalis*)
Goldenseal (*Hydrastis canadensis*)
Chaparral (*Larrea tridentata*)
Burdock (*Arctium lappa*)
Parsley Root (*Petroselinum crispum*)
Lobelia (*Lobelia inflata*)
Cayenne (*Capsicum spp.*)

This formula opens up the sinuses, stops infections, and cleanses the sinus area. Because many sinus related problems are systemic reactions that affect the entire body, gentle blood cleansing herbs were added to this formula.

Slumber

Valerian (*Valeriana officinalis*)
Passion Flower (*Passiflora incarnata*)
Mullein (*Verbascum thapsus*)
Hops (*Humulus lupulus*)
Lavender (*Lavandula angustifolia*)
Lobelia (*Lobelia inflata*)
Black Cohosh (*Cimicifuga racemosa*)
Blue Cohosh (*Caulophyllum thalictroides*)

This formula helps the body relax, relieves tension and prepares the body for a natural slumber.

Smoke Out

Wild Oats (*Avena sativa*)

Lobelia (*Lobelia inflata*)
Rose Hips (*Rosa spp.*)
Cayenne (*Capsicum spp.*)

This herbal formula helps reduce the desire for tobacco. The lobeline content of lobelia is similar to nicotine but is non-addictive and non-stimulating. The wild oats calm the nerves and the rose hips and cayenne support the body nutritionally.

Stings and Bites Ointment (Plantain ointment)

Plantain (*Plantago major*)
Bee s wax and olive oil base

Plantain has been used for centuries to ease the discomfort of bites and stings. Plantain draws toxins out from this skin while it soothes and reduces swelling. Plantain was used by Dr. Christopher to draw out infection from wounds that were not healed properly.

Stomach Comfort Formula, Kid-e-Col (Catnip and Fennel Combination)

Catnip (*Nepeta cataria*)
Fennel (*Foeniculum vulgare*)

This formula helps ease minor stomach discomfort associated with indigestion and bloating. This formula works well for colic, teething pain, flatulence, spasms, etc. A few drops of this formula (in glycerine form) may be placed on the pacifier of an upset or cranky infant.

Stop-Ache

White Willow (*Salix alba*)
Feverfew (*Tanacetum parthenium*)
Cloves (*Syzygium aromaticum*)
Valerian (*Valeriana officinalis*)
Wild Lettuce (*Lactuca quercina*)
Hops (*Humulus lupulus*)
Wood Betony (*Stachys officinales*)
Lobelia (*Lobelia inflata*)

This formula aids the body in reducing pain, inflamation and irritability associated with muscle soreness and headaches.

Super Garlic Immune Formula (Anti-Plague Formula)

Garlic (*Allium sativum*)
Comfrey (*Symphytum officinale*)
Replaced with Aloe Vera gel powder (*Aloe vera*) and Plantain (*Plantago major*)
Wormwood (*Artemisia absinthium*)
Lobelia (*Lobelia inflata*)
Marshmallow (*Althea officinalis*)
Oak Bark (*Quercus alba*)
Black Walnut (*Juglans nigra*)
Mullein (*Verbascum thapsus*)
Skullcap (*Scutellaria laterifloria*)
Uva Ursi (*Arctostaphylos uva ursi*)
In an apple cider vinegar, glycerine, honey base

This all purpose anti-biotic formula is used to treat colds, flus, congestion, infection, and all communicable diseases. It may be used in small amounts (one tablespoon three times a day) as a tonic during cold and flu season, or in large amounts (one tablespoon every hour) to fight off infection. This formula was designed by Dr. Christopher to treat bacterial and viral plagues.

Super-Lax

Aloe (*Aloe vera*)
Senna (*Senna alexandrina*)
Cascara Sagrada (*Rhamnus purshiana*)
Gentian (*Gentiana lutea*)
Ginger (*Zingiber officinale*)
Garlic (*Allium sativum*)
Cayenne (*Capsicum spp.*)
Turkey Rhubarb (*Rheum officinales*)
Flax Seed (*Linum usitatissimum*)

This formula cleanses, strengthens and nourishes the lower bowel. It is stronger than The Lower Bowel Formula but not as strong as the Quick Colon Cleanse Formula #1.

Thyroid Maintenance Formula (Kelp-T)

Parsley (*Petroselinum crispum*)
Watercress *(Nasturtium officinale*)
Kelp (*Ascophyllum nodosum*)
Mullein (*Verbascum thapsus*)
Nettle (*Urtica dioica*)
Irish Moss (*Chondrus crispus*)
Sheep Sorrel (*Rumex acetosella*)
Iceland Moss (*Cetraria islandica*)

The thyroid is located in the neck. It produces hormones that regulate metabolism, and growth. When the thyroid malfunctions, many diseases may result including goiter, hyperthyroidism, and hypothyroidism. This formula supports the proper function of the thyroid and parathyroid glands. It may be used with the Glandular System Formula (mullein and lobelia) either in capsule, fomentation, ointment, or oil forms.

Valerian Nerve Formula (Wild Lettuce and Valerian Combination)

Wild Lettuce (*Lactuca serriola*)
Valerian (*Valeriana officinalis*)

This formula is to be taken orally or massaged externally for relief of minor pain. It is a natural sedative, quiet and soothing to the nerves.

Vitalerbs and Kid-e-Mins

Alfalfa (*Medicago sativa*)
Dandelion (*Taraxacum officinale*)
Kelp (*Ascophyllum nodosum*)
Purple Dulce (*Rhodymenia palmetta*)
Spirulina (*Spirulina platensis*)
Irish Moss (*Chondrus crispus*)
Rose Hips (*Rosa canina*)
Beet (*Beta vulgaris rubra*)
Nutritional Yeast
Cayenne (*Capsicum spp.*)
Blue Violet (*Viola odorata*)
Oat Straw (*Avena sativa*)
Carrot Juice (*Daucus carota*)

Ginger (*Zingiber officinale*)
Barley Grass Juice (*Hordeum vulgare*)
Wheat Grass Juice (*Triticum spp.*)

This formula is a nature balanced, whole food vitamin and mineral supplement and an organic source of vitamins and minerals that are easy to assimilate because they are whole foods. The Vitalerbs formula is safe for all ages and may be taken during pregnancy or nursing.

X-Ceptic Tincture and Kid-e-Cep

Oak Bark (*Quercus alba*)
Goldenseal (*Hydrastis canadensis*)
Myrrh Gum (*Commiphora myrrha*)
Comfrey (*Symphytum officinale*)
Garlic (*Allium sativum*)
Cayenne (*Capsicum spp.*)

This tincture belongs in every first aid kit. It is used to fight infection, both externally and internally. It may also be used as a gargle or mouthwash for throat or tooth infections.

BIBLIOGRAPHY

Caster, Gladys B. A Comparison of Mother s Milk and Cow s Milk.

Christopher, John R. Regenerative Diet. Christopher Publications, P.O. Box 412, Springville UT 84663

Christopher, John R. School of Natural Healing. Christopher Publications, P.O. Box 412, Springville UT 84663

Dorland, W. A. Newman. The American Illustrated Medical Dictionary. Philadelphia & London: W. B. Saunders Co., 1947

Ehret, Arnold. Mucusless Diet Healing System. First published in 1922, enlarged and reprinted in 1953. Ehret Literature Publ. Co., Beaumont, California 92223.

Ellis, William E. The Healthview Newsletter, Number 14. 612 Rio Road West, Box 6670, Charlottesville, Virginia 22906.

Hyman, Harold Thomas. Handbook of Differential Diagnosis. Philadelphia, London: J. B. Lippincott Co.

Ingham, Eunice D. Stories the Feet Can Tell. Published by Eunice D. Ingham, P.O. Box 948, Rochester, New York 14603, 1938.

Jensen, B. The Joy of Living. Santa Barbara, California: J. F. Rowney Press, 1946.

Kellogg, John Harvey. Colon Hygiene. Battle Creek, Michigan: Modern Medicine Publishing Co.

Kervran, Louis. Biological Transmutations. Translated by Michael Abehsera. Swan House Publishing Co., P.O. Box 638, Binghamton, New York, 1972.

Kirschner, H. E., M.D. Nature s Healing Grasses. H. C. White Publications, P.O. Box 8014, Riverside, California 92505, 1960.

Kloss, Jethro. Back to Eden. Back to Eden Publishing Co.,PO Box 1439 Loma Linda, CA 92354, 1992

Kulvinskas, Viktoras. Survival into 21st Century. Omongod Press, P.O. Box 255, Wethersfield, Connecticut 06106.

Littlegreen, Inc. Transfiguration Diet. Christopher Publications, P.O. Box 412, Springville UT 84663

Mousert, Otto. Herbs. Eugene, Oregon: Elain M. Muhr, 1974.

Ott, John N. Health and Light. Original publisher: Devin-Adair Co., One Park Ave., Old Greenwich, Connecticut 06870, 1973.

Scott, Cyril. Folk Remedies.

Shook, Edward E. Advanced Treatise in Herbology.

Shook, Edward. Dr. E. Shook s Elementary Treatise in Herbology. Southland Books, Inc., 2717 7th Ave S., Birmingham, AL 35233

Taber, Clarence Wilbur. Taber s Cyclopedic Medical Dictionary. Philadelphia: F. A. Davis Co.

Tracy, Michael. The Mild Food Cook

Vogel, H. C. Alfred. The Nature Doctor. Verlag, Switzerland: Baiforce.

Walker, N. W. Diet and Salad Suggestions. Norwalk Press, 107 N. Cortez - suite 200, Prescott, AZ 86301.

Walker, N. W. Fresh Vegetable & Fruit Juices. Norwalk Press, 107 N. Cortez - suite 200, Prescott, AZ 86301.

Index

Bold entries indicate the primary listings for each formula

A

B

C

D

E

F

G

H

L

M

N

O

P

Q

R

S

T

U

V

W

X

Y

Z

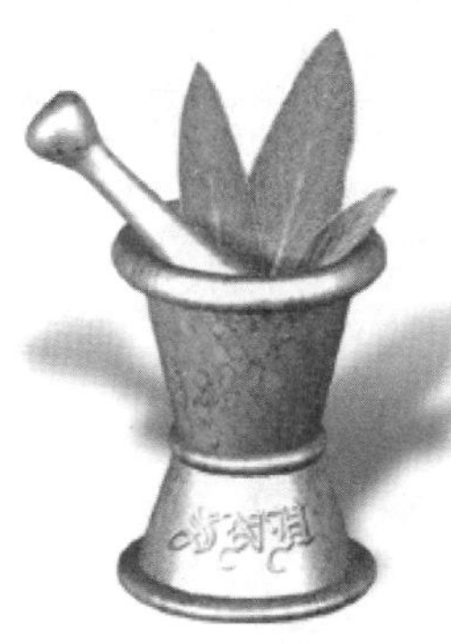

Dr. Christopher's
The School of Natural Healing

College of Herbal Studies

Outstanding Education Since 1953

Herbal Education

The School of Natural Healing was founded in 1953 by Dr. John R. Christopher and has been the means for thousands of students to begin and further their herbal knowledge and wisdom.

Few things are as rewarding and satisfying as being able to care for your own and your family's health. There is no safer avenue than herbal and natural healing, yet many people become overwhelmed at the prospect of herbal study towards becoming their own healer.

The School of Natural Healing's Master Herbalist Program will show you that you can become your own doctor, and that it is not as difficult as you may think. In as little as an hour a day, you could become a qualified healer and teacher in less than two years—all in the comfort of your own home.

Our courses are designed to teach herbalism from the ground up, beginning with foundational understandings of natural methodologies, and progressing through the many aspects of herbal healing, including herb identification, horticulture, medicinal usages, methods of preparation, and more. Students who complete the Master Herbalist Program are prepared to take care of both themselves and their families, and to share their knowledge and wisdom in the service of educating others.

Our School curriculum and philosophy is built upon the understanding and practice of four fundamental principles.

1. **Preventative Nutrition**
2. **Eradicating the Cause of Disease**
3. **Healing the Body through Natural Methods**
4. **Education**

Whether your interest is in a particular skill or in certification, The School of Natural Healing has courses to fit your needs

The Family Herbalist Program (Level 100)

The School's Family Herbalist Course is designed to empower you with the knowledge and confidence needed to tackle almost any health issue. The Family Herbalist Course is essential for anyone who wants to take charge of their own health and become more informed, educated, and independent. This course explores important concepts in natural medicine that even the most experienced natural healers need to know for success.

The Nutritional Herbalist Program (Levels 200-500)

The Nutritional Herbologist Program will instruct you to recognize, understand, and assist the body's inherent healing power. You will learn preventative medicine through the study of basic principles of natural healing. These courses focus on cause of disease, nutrition, elimination therapies, and herbal cleansing for the entire system. Training also includes the proper application of wholesome herbs and simple therapies. Using Dr. Christopher's world-famous herbal combinations and single herbs, you will learn how to cleanse, nourish, and build the body. Prerequisite: Family Herbalist Program

The Herbalist Program (Levels 600-1300)

In the Herbalist Program you will build upon the Nutritional Herbologist training with in-depth instruction in the use of herbal therapy to remove the cause of disease. Within these courses you help fulfill The School's mission to see a competent natural healer in every home. You will learn how to use the natural medicines that surround you with regional materials. In this program you will learn herb identification, selection, harvesting, horticulture, usage, herbal formulation and preparation. With enough materials to create your own herbal library, this program includes 18 hours of herbal therapy instruction from Dr. Christopher himself. A certificate of "Herbalist" is awarded upon completion of the first thirteen levels of the home study program.

The Advanced Herbalist Program (Levels 1400-2200)

The final nine courses of the Master Herbalist Program give you the skills to become a qualified teacher of herbology. As more people seek natural health, the need for competent educators increases in a variety of health related areas. The Advanced Herbalist Program provides the training to place you on the highest level of herbal competency. As a Master Herbalist you can teach others, so that they are able to take responsibility for their own health. The course study and preliminary examinations are administered through correspondence and provide instruction from the highest-qualified herbal practitioners and herbal pharmacists in the field. The final examinations are only administered at the Master Herbalist Certification Seminar, held at our facilities. This seminar gives you the opportunity of fine-tuning your skills with the clinical experience of some of the best herbalists in the country.

Help By Phone

Herbalists and Master Herbalists are available to students for tutorial and study aid by toll-free phone from 10:00 am to 4:00 pm MT Monday - Friday (1-800-372-8255). Master Herbalist David Christopher accepts calls from the general public Monday—Thursday between 1:00 pm and 2:00 pm MT. These calls are limited to 3 minutes each and are for educational instruction only.

Other Services

The School of Natural Healing provides a number of additional educational services and courses:

- Iridology Home Study Courses with David J. Pesek, Ph.D.
- Home Reflexology Course
- Aromatherapy Course
- Seminars with SNH instructors and Master Herbalists in your area.
- Monthly subscriptions to *A Healthier You* Audio Newsletter.
- Texts available on CD Rom for Windows.

For information on any of these services, please call or write to:

Iridology, A Wholistic Approach

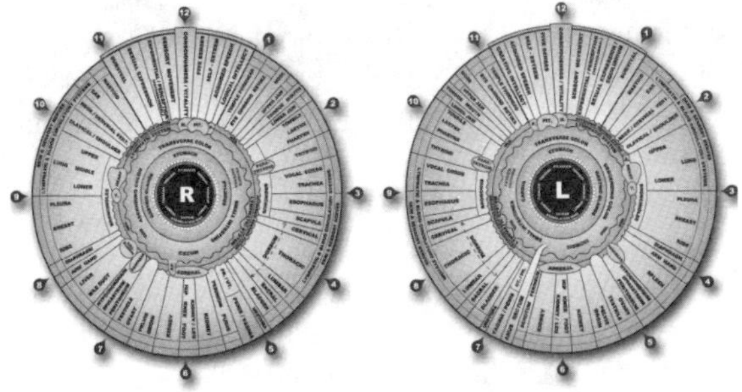

Two Level Iridology Home Study Course & Live Seminar

Dr. John R. Christopher utilized the science of Iridology thoughout his practice, and he had a tremendous appreciation for its benefits and usefulness in assessing health conditions in the body.

The School of Natural Healing has offered iridology study in the past with various teachers, however, in becoming acquainted with Dr. David J. Pesek, we found his understanding and methodology to be the foremost among his contemporaries. Though the mutual cooperation of Dr. Pesek and The School of Natural Healing, we know that we are offering the most comprehensive Iridology course available in North America.

This comprehensive, two level home study program and live seminar offers a fully informative and detailed look at the science and practice of Iridology. Beginning at basic levels and moving forward to advanced understandings of this art and science, the student will gain a powerful knowledge of revealing levels of health, inflammation and degeneration within the human body, along with thought and emotional patterns.

Call now to find out more about this amazing science.

The School of Natural Healing

1-800-372-8255

The Complete Herbal Writings of Dr. John R. Christopher

on CD Rom for Windows

Includes the full texts of:

School of Natural Healing
Every Woman's Herbal
Herbal Home Health Care
Over 6 years of Dr. Christopher's Newsletters
Over 2,000 pages of previously unpublished writings
Over 200 illustrations and photos of herbs

Also includes color pictures of nearly 100 herbs

This Folio® based program can allow you to search quickly and easily for any word or topic Dr. Christopher ever wrote about. Search in a particular book or scan the entire library. This easy-to-use CD Rom will speed up your study and research time.

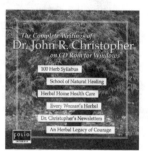

(This disk may not work on all versions of Windows)

Only $98.95

A Healthier You Audio Newsletter 1 Year Subscription

These informative audio cassettes are select recordings of Master Herbalist David Christopher's popular radio program "A Healthier You." Each 60 minute cassette offers up-to-date information and common sense regarding a variety of health topics, herbs, natural treatments and therapies.

Only $39.95
Audio Newsletter Back-Issues Available
Look for our list of back-issue titles of cassettes. Single tapes or volumes of 12 are available.

Dr. John. R. Christopher's
Natural Healing Newsletters
Back - Issues

Begun as a monthly newsletter in 1980, these various treatises are available in single issuses and in volumes of 12.

Herbal Facts
Information
Case Histories
Recipes
Testimonials
Formulas
and More!

Volume 1 Nos. 1 - 12 item #95150
Volume 2 Nos. 1 - 12 item #95250
Volume 3 Nos. 1 - 12 item #95350
Volume 4 Nos. 1 - 12 item #95450
Volume 5 Nos. 1 - 12 item #95550
Volume 6 Nos. 1 - 12 item #95650

#95100	Vol. 1 Intro	There Are No Incurable Diseases
#95101	Vol. 1 No. 1	Does Your Colon Feed or Poison You?
#95102	Vol. 1 No. 2	The Blood Stream: River of Life
#95103	Vol. 1 No. 3	The Ten Most Important Herbs
#95104	Vol. 1 No. 4	The Dairy King
#95105	Vol. 1 No. 5	Let Not Your Heart Be Troubled
#95106	Vol. 1 No. 6	Pancreas Panacea
#95107	Vol. 1 No. 7	Women's New Lease on Life
#95108	Vol. 1 No. 8	Bone, Flesh & Cartilage
#95109	Vol. 1 No. 9	Infection - The Killer
#95110	Vol. 1 No. 10	Why Distilled Water?
#95111	Vol. 1 No. 11	How Important is Calcium?
#95112	Vol. 1 No. 12	Cayenne, Part 1
#95201	Vol. 2 No. 1	Afraid of Frayed Nerves - Nerves Part 1
#95202	Vol. 2 No. 2	Cell Deterioration
#95203	Vol. 2 No. 3	Adrenals
#95204	Vol. 2 No. 4	Chocolate - America's Foremost Addiction
#95205	Vol. 2 No. 5	The RH Factor
#95206	Vol. 2 No. 6	Meat Freaks (or Hanging on the Meat Hook)
#95207	Vol. 2 No. 7	Sundae Mourning - A Short Treatise on Ice Cream
#95208	Vol. 2 No. 8	How Efficient is our Eyesight?
#95209	Vol. 2 No. 9	Garlic: Man's Best Friend in a Toxic World
#95210	Vol. 2 No. 10	Oak Bark
#95211	Vol. 2 No. 11	Nervous in the Service - Nerves Part 2
#95212	Vol. 2 No. 12	Alfalfa - The Fodder of All Foods

#95301	Vol. 3 No. 1	Herbal First Aid - Part 1
#95302	Vol. 3 No. 2	Herbal First Aid - Part 2
#95303	Vol. 3 No. 3	Licorice - The Legendary Herb
#95304	Vol. 3 No. 4	Chaparral - The Governor's Herb
#95305	Vol. 3 No. 5	Importance of Fresh Juices
#95306	Vol. 3 No. 6	Men's Diseases - Part 1
#95307	Vol. 3 No. 7	Herbs in Pregnancy & Childbirth - Part 1
#95308	Vol. 3 No. 8	Herbs in Pregnancy & Childbirth - Part 2
#95309	Vol. 3 No. 9	The Breath of Life
#95310	Vol. 3 No. 10	Men's Diseases - Part 2
#95311	Vol. 3 No. 11	Arthritis - A Needless Crippler
#95312	Vol. 3 No. 12	Back to Nature
#95401	Vol. 4 No. 1	Cold, Flu, and Related Nuisances
#95402	Vol. 4 No. 2	Needless Surgery
#95403	Vol. 4 No. 3	Curative Comfrey
#95404	Vol. 4 No. 4	Dr. John R. Christopher - A Memorial
#95405	Vol. 4 No. 5	Pain Palliatives
#95406	Vol. 4 No. 6	Now Hear This! - Ear Remedies
#95407	Vol. 4 No. 7	Ten Honorable Herbs
#95408	Vol. 4 No. 8	On Digestion
#95409	Vol. 4 No. 9	Oriental Herbs
#95410	Vol. 4 No. 10	European Herbs
#95411	Vol. 4 No. 11	American Indian Herbs
#95412	Vol. 4 No. 12	Our Healing Vegetables & Seasonings
#95501	Vol. 5 No. 1	Let's Make Our Foods be Our Medicines...
#95502	Vol. 5 No. 2	Historical Botanicals - Part 1
#95503	Vol. 5 No. 3	Historical Botanicals - Part 2
#95504	Vol. 5 No. 4	Barberry
#95505	Vol. 5 No. 5	Bayberry
#95506	Vol. 5 No. 6	Black Cohosh
#95507	Vol. 5 No. 7	Black Walnut
#95508	Vol. 5 No. 8	Blessed Thistle
#95509	Vol. 5 No. 9	Blue Cohosh
#95510	Vol. 5 No. 10	Blue Vervain
#95511	Vol. 5 No. 11	Buckthorn
#95512	Vol. 5 No. 12	Burdock
#95601	Vol. 6 No. 1	Cascara Sagrada
#95602	Vol. 6 No. 2	Catnip
#95603	Vol. 6 No. 3	Cayenne - Part 2
#95604	Vol. 6 No. 4	Cedar
#95605	Vol. 6 No. 5	Chickweed
#95606	Vol. 6 No. 6	Cloves
#95607	Vol. 6 No. 7	Cramp Bark
#95608	Vol. 6 No. 8	Eyebright
#95609	Vol. 6 No. 9&10	Lobelia
#95611	Vol. 6 No. 11	Dandelion
#95612	Vol. 6 No. 12	Echinacea
#95701	Vol. 7 No. 1	Fennel
#95702	Vol. 7 No. 2	Flaxseed
#95703	Vol. 7 No. 3	Ginger